# THE NEW
# Eating Right
## FOR A BAD GUT

*The Complete Nutritional
Guide to Ileitis, Colitis,
Crohn's Disease, and
Inflammatory Bowel Disease*

## James Scala, Ph.D.

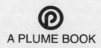

A PLUME BOOK

PLUME
Published by the Penguin Group
Penguin Putnam Inc., 375 Hudson Street, New York, New York 10014, U.S.A.
Penguin Books Ltd, 27 Wrights Lane, London W8 5TZ, England
Penguin Books Australia Ltd, Ringwood, Victoria, Australia
Penguin Books Canada Ltd, 10 Alcorn Avenue, Toronto, Ontario, Canada M4V 3B2
Penguin Books (N.Z.) Ltd, 182–190 Wairau Road, Auckland 10, New Zealand

Penguin Books Ltd, Registered Offices: Harmondsworth, Middlesex, England

This revised edition published by Plume, a member of Penguin Putnam Inc.
Original edition published by NAL Books as *Eating Right for a Bad Gut*.

First Printing (Revised Edition), March, 2000
10  9  8  7  6  5  4

 REGISTERED TRADEMARK—MARCA REGISTRADA

LIBRARY OF CONGRESS CATALOGING-IN-PUBLICATION DATA:

Scala, James.
    The new eating right for a bad gut : the complete nutritional
guide to ileitis, colitis, Crohn's disease, and inflammatory bowel
disease / James Scala.
        p.   cm.
    ISBN 0-452-27976-3
    1. Inflammatory bowel diseases—Diet therapy.   I. Title.
RC862.I53S234   2000
616.3'440654—dc21                                    99-38609
                                                        CIP

Printed in the United States of America
Set in New Baskerville
Designed by Leonard Telesca

# Contents

## Good Nutrition—The Best Medicine

People suffering from IBD, Crohn's disease, and other disorders require more protein (in fish, fowl, and vegetables), less animal fat, more good fat (olive and flax oil, avocados), and additional calories from complex natural carbohydrates (fruits, vegetables, grains, and pastas) to help prevent flare-ups. This completely revised and updated edition of *Eating Right for a Bad Gut* explores the nutritional challenges sufferers face and how these often debilitating symptoms can be relieved.

### Discover:

- Which foods are taboo—and why
- Who is at greater risk for IBD
- "Safe foods"
- Tips on reading labels
- The crucial role of potassium and other minerals
- How to combat serious flare-ups with predigested formula diets that give your digestive tract a rest
- Strategies to shift your dietary fat balance and reduce all animal fat

. . . and more

Coping with IBD and other abdominal disorders begins with good food selection, sensible supplementation, and ongoing stress management. With this indispensable guide, you'll learn how to tame your "bad gut" and live a more pain-free, abundant life.

"Offers ways to get lasting relief through proper diet, exercise, and stress management."
—*Rocky Mountain News*

DR. JAMES SCALA is a certified nutritional specialist. His professional life has spanned many areas, including research, teaching, corporate management, lecturing, and writing. He has been the nutritionist for the U.S. Olympic Ski Team, the Voyager flight, and three Mt. Everest expeditions. He is the author of *The New Arthritis Relief Diet, The High Blood Pressure Relief Diet, Prescription for Longevity,* and *Look 10 Years Younger, Feel 10 Years Better.*

**Also by Dr. James Scala**

*The New Arthritis Relief Diet*
*The High Blood Pressure Relief Diet*
*Prescription for Longevity*

# Acknowledgments

Many people with bowel disorders will benefit from the teachings in this book. My interviews with them taught me that the human spirit knows no challenge it cannot overcome. To them I will always be grateful for the lessons learned.

No book is possible without an agent who believes in and supports the author; Al Zuckerman is that agent.

Behind the book is a supportive, patient editor who knows the audience; that is Deborah Brody.

Nancy, my wife and best friend, also joins me in acknowledging the support of all these people and we dedicate the work to them.

# Preface

*"Let Food Be Thy Medicine"*
—Hippocrates, c. 450 B.C.

## The Iniquity of Chronic Illness

Crohn's disease and other inflammatory bowel diseases (IBD) are chronic illnesses, meaning you will always have them even when they're in remission (not active). Thus IBD has many things in common with rheumatoid arthritis and other inflammatory diseases, in that all are characterized by periods of inactivity when life is pretty normal, interspersed with active periods called flare-ups when you're feeling pretty miserable. With IBD, such flare-ups are accompanied by pain and diarrhea, so the main objective is to get the disease back into remission.

My objective in this book is to help those of you with an inflammatory bowel disease establish dietary and lifestyle habits that are least likely to cause flare-ups. In this way you can make subsequent flare-ups as mild as possible, keep IBD in remission, and achieve a more abundant life.

## Inflammation of IBD

All inflammatory diseases share one common characteristic: inflammation. Many, such as Crohn's disease, are also autoimmune diseases, which means some components of the immune system attack the body's own tissues. Fortunately, this immune attack is set in motion by inflammation, so your strategy should be simple: stop inflammation and keep it from starting—and if it does, keep it as mild as possible.

Later chapters will explain how diet can reduce inflammation and provide effective dietary plans to support your efforts.

## Diet Can Reduce Medication

Similar to any chronic illness, IBD often, but not always, requires daily medication. Unfortunately, this lulls many people into believing that medication is the only way to treat IBD, so they throw diet and lifestyle to the wind. That is wrong! Diet is even more important when any medication (especially daily medication) is required. In fact, when correctly and consistently followed, diet can reduce the need for such medication. Clinical studies have shown that the need is reduced by 70 percent in some cases, meaning certain people will never have to take any medication, while many others will be able to get by with less.

## What Is IBD?

Inflammatory bowel disease (IBD) is the name given to diseases that cause the bowel wall to become inflamed. Your doctor may call the disease by a number of terms, such as colitis, proctitis, enteritis, or ileitis; however, you'll probably be told you have ulcerative colitis, colitis, Crohn's disease, or a combination of them. For our purposes, we will call all of these diseases IBD. I urge you to purchase both of the books listed in the references for this preface (all references for each chapter are at the end of the book). They explain very clearly the problems you must deal with.

*Ulcerative colitis* is an IBD with ulcers, open sores, and inflammation of the large intestine. It almost always causes bloody, watery stools and involves the rectum. Ulcerative colitis can involve most of the large intestine beginning at the anus. When the entire organ is involved, there are seldom any areas that aren't inflamed and ulcerated. Plain *colitis* doesn't involve ulcerations and seems to be confined more to the upper part of the large intestine. When it's found adjacent to the ileum (the lower portion of the small intestine), it's sometimes called *Crohn's colitis.*

*Crohn's disease* is characterized by inflammation that spreads deep into the bowel wall and is usually confined to one or more segments of the small intestine, especially the ileum. In about 50 percent of cases, it includes both the ileum and the first part of the large intestine, the colon. About 20 percent of cases involve only the colon.

## Symptoms of IBD

Whether it involves the large or small intestine, IBD produces diarrhea and serious abdominal pain. Both Crohn's disease and colitis frequently cause rectal bleeding, while ulcerative colitis often causes serious bleeding. Persistent loss of blood can lead to anemia, or a shortage of red blood cells, because red blood cells are lost faster than your body can make them.

Intestinal inflammation can result in poor absorption of nutrients, and the diarrhea causes an actual loss of nutrients, especially minerals, through the stools. Together, these symptoms can cause weight loss and poor nutrition; in young people, they can even slow growth. Persistent intestinal inflammation can require aggressive medical nutrition treatment, because the patient can actually be starving to death. While it seems impossible for starvation to happen in a modern society with such obvious abundance, it can occur in these patients because their intestinal tracts are not working. In addition, they avoid food because it causes severe pain, discomfort, and even bloody stools.

IBD is often characterized by other symptoms that precede the intestinal flare-up. These warning signs include one

or more small canker sores in the mouth; inflammation of
the eyes; inflammation of a joint, such as a knee or a wrist;
and ulcerlike sores and red nodules on the skin, especially
on the abdomen and legs and even on the head. Although
the red nodules aren't painful and the canker sores are simply irksome, the ulcers can become infected.

## Flare-ups: The Gut Gets Angry!

IBD can go into remission for years, especially if you follow an appropriate diet, even though you may always seem to
have watery stools unless you can control this symptom with
dietary fiber. During these long quiescent periods, life seems
normal except for occasional diarrhea, which is a minor discomfort compared with other aspects of the disease.

The return of IBD with all its symptoms is called a flare-up.
The term *flare-up* covers a wide range of symptoms, from abdominal cramps and diarrhea to the need for hospitalization. It can be serious enough that total parenteral nutrition
(TPN) is required, meaning the patient is fed through a
major vein and the digestive system is completely bypassed.
One of my objectives is to help people with IBD learn how to
identify and eliminate foods that cause flare-ups.

Research has confirmed that sensible diet and supplements
can help IBD go into remission and remain that way. (Some
studies indicate remission can last for years.) These findings
are consistent with the extensive research scientists have done
on rheumatoid arthritis (a more common inflammatory disease) and multiple sclerosis, which proved that both of these
diseases are improved by a correct diet and sensible omega-3
oil supplements. Another of my objectives is to help you understand these oils and how to use them to your advantage.

References to medical research journals appear on pages
265–68; their purpose is to help you face down the skeptics,
so the notion that diet can't help will simply disappear. If
you'd like further information, these references will help
you get started in a medical library.

*Examples of How Diet Can Help Manage Chronic Disease*

- Diabetics must take insulin every day. They can reduce insulin intake to a minimum if they follow a diet rich in complex carbohydrates and fiber.
- Hypertension (high blood pressure) can be controlled by medication. Hypertensives can also reduce their medication by about 85 percent through diet alone.
- Rheumatoid arthritis and its variations can't be cured, not even by the "right" diet. However, diet can minimize inflammation and reduce medication up to 70 percent—and make life much better.
- Paraplegics can improve the quality of their lives by good dietary management. Inactivity causes them to get bladder infections; a diet that produces high levels of benzoic acid in the urine prevents this. It calls for eating benzoic acid–producing foods such as cranberries or a variation called cloudberries.
- Gout, a buildup of uric acid in the system, can be treated more effectively by diet than by medication. Medication is the treatment of last resort.
- Multiple sclerosis, an inflammatory autoimmune disease that attacks the nerves, can often be significantly helped by diet. Yes, the diet is spartan, but the results are worth the sacrifice.

Many other examples illustrate how good diet planning can improve your quality of life when you have a chronic illness. Good diet can't possibly make the illness worse, and clinical research and experience prove it can help a great deal—so why not give it a try?

## Basics

To gain a better understanding of IBD, we need to build a common language. This calls for a brief review of the digestive system and some characteristics of the disease. I suggest that as you read you write questions in the margins or on a sheet of paper. They will probably be answered later in the book, but if they aren't, write to me and I guarantee I'll answer, even if it is to say "I don't know" or "Nobody knows." Also, be sure to consult the books listed in the references for this preface (page 265).

## The Small Intestine

Digestion begins in the mouth. When we chew our food, we mix it with saliva, a lubricant that helps to break down starches. Chewing also breaks food into small pieces, increasing its surface area, so the fluids and digestive enzymes of the stomach and small intestine can break it down into protein, fat, carbohydrate, dietary fiber, and a number of vitamins and minerals. (Enzymes are proteins that our body makes to carry out specific functions. The enzymes made by the stomach are for digesting food.) After that, the partially digested food leaves the stomach and enters the intestines.

Extending almost 20 feet, the small intestine is actually three organs. The upper part, the *duodenum,* is where most of the digestion of food really occurs. Here, thanks to the pancreas (which makes and passes the digestive enzymes into the duodenum), protein, fat, and carbohydrates are completely broken down into their simplest chemical building blocks. (I'll explain these building blocks in other chapters.) At the same time, bile acids produced in the liver are passed into the gallbladder and through the bile duct into the duodenum. In a way, bile acids are natural human soaps (detergents) that help mix fats with water so the pancreatic enzymes can digest them.

The middle section of the small intestine, the *jejunum,* is where the food is completely digested and nutrients are absorbed into the blood.

After the jejunum comes the *ileum.* Absorption continues here, but the solid material entering this section is mostly nondigestible food residue and will pass from the ileum through a valve into the large intestine, the next part of the bowel. Food spends about four hours going from the mouth to the ileum where, if everything is normal, it's reduced mostly to water, dissolved minerals, and undigested plant residue called dietary fiber. Passage through the entire small intestine takes from one to two hours. Food is moved by the muscles in the intestinal wall, which squeeze the food along in a wavelike motion called peristalsis. Thus, the digestive system is like a long sorting vat where food is reduced to its simplest chemical subunits, which either enter the blood or exit the system.

## The Large Intestine

The large intestine consists of four sections: the *ascending colon, transverse colon, descending colon,* and *sigmoid colon.* Water and minerals are exchanged in the ascending and transverse sections. ("Exchanged" means that they are absorbed into the body from the intestinal contents.) Under some conditions, water is also released into the intestine and increases the water content of the stool. This passing of water into the intestine can also include the loss of minerals such as potassium and calcium.

Microorganisms live in the large intestine, and their function is to break down the undigestible residue in food and dietary fiber even more. This natural process produces some important by-products and converts the residue to a paste we call the stool. In the process, intestinal bacteria actually produce about half our vitamin K need. The last section of the intestine, the sigmoid colon, connects to the anus and consists of a series of valves and baffles that help to move the stool along. The anus is itself a valve connecting the digestive system to the external environment.

If you want more detailed information on the bowel and its functions, read *Your Gut Feelings,* as well as literature published by the National Foundation for Crohn's and Colitis (386 Park Avenue South, 17th Floor, New York, NY 10016-8804; (800) 932-2423).

## A Nutritionist's View of an Inflamed Bowel

An inflamed bowel is similar to any inflamed tissue. A bruised or sprained joint is swollen and/or stiff, hurts when it's moved, and is sensitive to touch and even temperature. A joint inflamed by arthritis hurts and doesn't work well. Drugs can help reduce the swelling and eliminate the pain, but rest is the best remedy for a swollen joint.

An inflamed bowel is also swollen. However, since it is a "tube" with a strong outer muscle wall, inflammation makes the central opening smaller. The diameter of a swollen small intestine can shrink to about an eighth of an inch in diameter, the width of a small drinking straw. Yet, in contrast to a swollen joint, it is almost impossible, without hospitalization, to fully rest the intestine. So, the simplest remedy—rest—is almost out of the question for the average outpatient. I say "almost" because some predigested drink mixes can be taken at home and work quite well in moderate cases.

When an inflamed intestine is called on to digest food, it hurts. Peristalsis, the normal motion during digestion, is simply too painful, like going up and down stairs with an inflamed joint.

An inflamed intestine is sensitive to both contact with undigested bits of food that have coarse edges and some food chemicals in spicy foods. When you eat, your body naturally produces bile acids that aren't a problem for a normal intestine. However, they can be painfully irritating to an inflamed intestine and accelerate diarrhea.

## Strictures: An Analogy to a Damaged Joint

An inflamed bowel can return to normal, but when it does, a stricture sometimes remains. A stricture is similar to the deformed scar tissue in an arthritic joint or the scar tissue left from a serious cut. In the small intestine, the scar tis-

sue can circle the intestine for a short distance in each direction, or it can be an entire area along the intestine.

Another mechanism can cause a stricture. Inflammation
results from the production of a material called a
prostaglandin (see Chapter Ten). Along with the inflammatory prostaglandin, other materials called leukotrienes are
produced that indirectly cause joint damage in arthritis. It is
almost certain that these leukotrienes do the same thing to
the intestine, since they show up at higher levels in people
with IBD. We'll discuss this in Chapter Ten and you will see
how diet can reduce them.

A stricture causes trouble because it's an unyielding area
in an otherwise homogeneous and smooth organ that undu-
lates in peristaltic motion. Because it's not as flexible, a stricture can't move with the surrounding tissue, so it "pulls"
when the intestine moves. Partially digested food can become stuck in a stricture, leading to a blockage that can be
painful; in severe cases, hospitalization is required to clear
the obstruction.

When a stricture is present, hard pieces of food, such as
bits of nuts, seeds of fruit, or even coarse, undigested bran
from cereal, can be irritating. That is why your vegetables
should be cooked until soft and shouldn't be fried, and why
apples, potatoes, and similar foods should be peeled.

## Emotions and IBD

Bowel and joint comparisons end with the emotions, unless a person suffers from rheumatoid arthritis, in which case
stress can cause flare-ups. Your entire digestive system is in-
tricately involved with emotions. Who hasn't felt a little sick
during times of extreme stress? We all know people who have
become so ill from stress or terrible thoughts that they vomit
or get diarrhea. I've seen people get sick while riding on a
merry-go-round or seeing a movie with lots of graphic gore.
Visual signals to the brain can trigger a major reaction in the
stomach and digestive system. Since the bowels respond to

emotions, it follows that emotional upset or stress can make inflamed bowels worse.

## The Psychology of IBD as Derived from Interviews

There does seem to be a psychological profile for people with IBD. Most of the patients I interviewed had difficulty dealing with emotions in childhood, many had an unsettling family life, and, as youths, their lives were characterized by emotional upset. However, I've also talked to IBD sufferers who are stable, joyful, and come from happy, nonstressful homes. This leads me to believe that a more significant factor is how they deal with stress.

Many people who get IBD simply don't deal well with stress. They say, "I just keep my mouth shut" or "There was no one to talk it out with." Even though this observation doesn't show cause and effect, it does indicate that the body responds to stress in various ways. Some people describe themselves as "professional internalizers," and I conclude that when faced with a tough situation, they don't "explode," they "implode." The stress stays inside!

One gastroenterologist who practices at a major university remarked: "Exam time is Crohn's time. Most of our diagnoses are made then, when the kids are under a lot of stress!" Another doctor showed me two letters from patients and said, "I can always identify the IBD patient." One patient's letter was written without respect for margins; the small careful writing went from edge to edge. Every square inch of paper was used. In contrast, the other letter looked quite normal, with regular writing within margins. The doctor said, "I can always spot the [patients with] intestinal disorders when they write me a letter. They're usually a variation of [the former]."

Although research confirms there is no psychological cause and effect for IBD, the emotions clearly have a major effect on the emergence and course of the disease. This be-

came obvious to me from the responses I got on a questionnaire I had prepared. When I asked what caused flare-ups,
every person with IBD mentioned variations on two things:
stress first and food second. Several creative people wrote
"stress" diagonally across the questionnaire and "food" on
the top and bottom.

On the same questionnaire, fatigue was often identified as
a cause of flare-ups. Fatigue can mean that someone is tired
from overwork, exercising too much, or not getting enough
rest or sleep. Poor nutrition and dietary habits, including excess caffeine consumption, also cause fatigue.

Some support groups use professional discussion leaders
to help people explore their emotions and learn how to deal
with stress. There's a solution to every problem. "Self-health
management" begins with good food selection, sensible supplementation, and ongoing stress control.

## What Causes IBD?

No one knows the exact cause of IBD, but the most prevalent theory puts it in the same league with other inflammatory diseases, such as rheumatoid arthritis. Inflammation is
actually a type of defense mounted by the body when a tissue
is attacked by a virus or something else. This theory teaches
that the inflammatory disease is initiated by a virus and accelerated when the immune system mistakenly attacks one
or several of its own tissues where the virus resides. In IBD,
the intestine is the target; in rheumatoid arthritis, it's the
joint tissue; in multiple sclerosis, it's the nerves. For a more
extensive discussion of this process, read my book *The New
Arthritis Relief Diet.*

## Who Gets IBD?

About 120,000 people in the United States are diagnosed
annually with IBD. An equal percentage of women and men
get it. Most are diagnosed between the ages of 15 and 30. In

about 25 percent of cases there's a family connection, but it's not clear whether the causes are genetic or environmental. Further research is needed to uncover this aspect of the disease.

## IBD in Children

About 20 percent of adults with IBD exhibited symptoms before age 15. The disease is rarely diagnosed before age 10 unless another family member has it. One major clue in children under age 4 is that they begin to fall behind peers in physical development, especially height. IBD is not easily diagnosed in children because it starts slowly and builds. Consequently, it's not uncommon for a pediatrician to think IBD is something else. Because of the symptoms, a doctor could justifiably suspect emotional problems as the cause of cramps or anorexia. For instance, a child with IBD associates food with discomfort; hence, he or she logically learns to be a picky eater and not to eat foods that cause pain. (If you ate and got sick, you'd cut back on eating, too.)

It is essential for children with IBD to get adequate nutrition, especially calories, so that their growth and development are not stunted. There are several excellent approaches to overcome this challenge. Supplemental foods for mild cases are listed in Chapter Eight. The next step may be enteral nutrition, in which alimental (predigested) food is tubed directly into the stomach. The last approach is total parenteral nutrition (TPN), in which nourishment is supplied directly into a large vein. All three approaches help to speed remission, avoid the use of steroids, and maintain growth.

## The Incidence of IBD Is Growing

In 1934, Dr. Burrill B. Crohn, an American physician, described an inflamed bowel; the condition became known as *Crohn's disease*. Thirty years later, the list of inflammatory diseases had grown. However, people with one of these diseases, especially children, often went from doctor to doctor searching for a diagnosis. Too often they were referred to a psychiatrist, with the idea that the symptoms were "in the head."

By 1994, IBD had become so common that local Sunday newspaper magazine supplements carried full-page advertisements for "ostomy" centers, where parts of the intestine are surgically removed from people who have IBD. This change in attitude is the best indication of how rapidly awareness of the seriousness of these diseases has grown.

# PART I

# Meeting the
# Challenges of IBD

Inflammatory bowel disease presents the patient and his or her family and friends with many challenges. While these challenges run the gamut from psychology to surgery, they can all be made more bearable by good diet and nutrition; in fact, just getting all the nutrients they need is difficult for people with bowel disorders.

Part I will acquaint you with the special nutritional challenges presented by IBD. Like any chronic disease, IBD has its own special requirements, and as a nutritional biochemist, I would like to help you address them to improve the quality of your life.

My second objective is to enlighten you on IBD's nutritional challenges and show you how they can be managed. I use the word *managed* instead of the word *solved* because a chronic illness is never cured. Consequently, the most realistic objective is to learn how to manage IBD so you can get on with your life. My aim is to help you achieve this goal so you can live a longer, more abundant life.

# CHAPTER 1

# *Nutritional Challenges for People with IBD*

You know when an inflamed intestine doesn't function correctly because it hurts and you have diarrhea—possibly bloody diarrhea. Particles of food eaten within twenty-four hours often appear in the watery stools, proving they weren't completely digested. These observations are the source of nutritional challenges in IBD.

## Malabsorption of Vitamins and Minerals

Malabsorption, literally "sick absorption," occurs during inflammation when absorption of nutrients is impaired or nonexistent. And it may even persist after the flare-up has subsided.

Malabsorption of specific vitamins and minerals depends upon where the small intestine is inflamed. Most vitamins and many minerals are absorbed throughout the small intestine, and some vitamins are even partially absorbed from the stomach. For example, the absorption of vitamin $B_{12}$ occurs in the lower 4 feet of the small intestine and depends on the secretion of an intrinsic factor by the stomach. Therefore, if the most severely inflamed portion is the terminal 4 feet, or if that portion has been removed, $B_{12}$ absorption is impaired or nonexistent, and the only means of meeting the

$B_{12}$ requirement is by injection. Likewise, some minerals, such as zinc, are absorbed from the large intestine; if it has been damaged or removed, a similar malabsorption problem exists, which can be solved by injection. Meeting the requirements for all other vitamins and minerals can be dealt with by a process chemists call *mass action,* and nutritionists call *supplementation.*

Mass action and its nutritional application, supplementation, are simple concepts you'll easily grasp. Think of your intestine as a long tube through which nutrients pass into the blood. The recommended daily intake (RDI) takes into account normal human absorption and other factors, and tells us how much of each nutrient we need to maintain good health.

Suppose you have malabsorption because of IBD, and that only about 60 percent of your normal absorption is working. We can apply some high-school algebra and correct the situation by supplementation; hence, malabsorption is a controllable challenge.

If you need "A" amount of a nutrient and you only absorb 60 percent because of IBD malabsorption, how much of the nutrient do you need to meet your special requirement? The solution is: $A = 0.6x$; by transposing terms, $x = A \div 0.6$. Suppose you're a 15-year-old girl and your calcium RDI is 1,000 milligrams daily. Substitute 1,000 milligrams for A in our equation. The answer is: $1,000 \div 0.6 = 1,667$ milligrams (rounded off), or about twice the RDI for calcium. You can use calcium-fortified orange juice (which also supplies potassium) and take calcium supplements (calcium citrate) to get at least 1,500 milligrams daily.

While calcium is a special nutrient that you can take as a calcium supplement, the same concept applies to the other nutrients, all of which can be put into two single tablets taken daily. The easiest way to solve the malabsorption challenge is to take one extra tablet daily. So, instead of taking two tablets which the label declares as a serving, take three to compensate for malabsorption.

Vitamin K is a special case. We rely on food for part of our vitamin K need and on intestinal microbes for the rest. Impaired absorption is likely to reduce the vitamin K absorbed from food; coupled with other intestinal problems, such as diarrhea, or removal of some of the intestine, we're likely not to get enough vitamin K—perhaps none—from our intestinal flora. This deficiency can cause bruises or excessive bleeding from cuts or scrapes; however, the deficiency may not show up until something serious happens. That's why it's important to raise the issue with your physician. A special vitamin K supplement can be prescribed to ensure that the problem never occurs.

Thanks to technology, we have the means to make up any nutrient shortfall with sensible supplements so that malabsorption does not have to lead to malnutrition.

## Consequences of Malabsorption

Failure to thrive (when a child falls behind in growth and development and lacks energy) is often seen in children with IBD since they usually don't eat enough, and the nutrients in their food aren't being absorbed. Consequently, they aren't getting enough calories and are probably falling a little short in protein, vitamins, and minerals.

Similar problems are seen in adults, but since men and women are no longer growing, they show up as an inability to maintain weight and a general lack of energy. Sometimes women with IBD don't maintain enough body fat and stop menstruating, a problem that can also arise from a lack of protein. Whatever the cause, the only solution is to get more calories from protein-rich and carbohydrate-rich foods, and to add the correct oils, such as olive and flax oils. Calories are discussed in more detail in Chapter Eighteen.

Other consequences of long-term malabsorption include all the nightmarish illnesses of vitamin and mineral deficiencies. In the beginning, these problems manifest as rather vague symptoms we all experience once in a while. Irritability and depression come first, but the most common, overt symptoms

are cracking of the lips at the corners of the mouth, poor lus-
ter of hair, weak or brittle fingernails, chills or feeling cold
easily, a lack of energy, and recurring headaches.

Don't we *all* experience these vague symptoms from time
to time? Of course we do! But if you have IBD and any of
these symptoms persist for days, you must see your doctor.
The best insurance against them is to use nutritional supplements, which come in many forms and can ensure good
nutrition.

## Table 1.1

### Common Symptoms of Minor Nutrient Deficiencies

| Symptom | Nutritional Deficit |
| --- | --- |
| Failure to thrive<br>Poor growth in children<br>Tiredness in adults<br>Muscle wasting | Insufficient calories, protein, and some micronutrients |
| Cold feeling, poor<br>complexion, tiredness, anemia | Iron and folic acid |
| Sore mouth, cracks at<br>corners of lips, sore tongue | B-complex of vitamins, especially folic acid |
| Loss of taste and smell<br>Cuts don't heal quickly<br>Postadolescent acne | Zinc |
| Mild depression<br>Confusion, irritability | B-complex of vitamins, especially folic acid |
| Muscle aches<br>Low back pain | Calcium and magnesium |
| Muscle weakness, spasm<br>Numbness and tingling | Electrolytes, especially potassium and possibly sodium |
| Bruises, cuts don't<br>heal quickly | Vitamin K and possibly vitamin C |

I've summarized the symptoms of deficiency in Table 1.1. As you look at this table, you may conclude that you've had every symptom. I can assure you that I have also had them, because they are the signs of many minor illnesses that include work-related stress, being overtired, and coming down with a cold or flu. The best medicine is prevention in the form of good nutrition.

## Special Challenges of Macronutrients

Macronutrients are nutrients we need in quantities measured in grams instead of milligrams or micrograms. They include protein (about 45 to 65 grams daily), carbohydrate (about 300 grams), and fat (about 55 grams). In contrast, most vitamins and minerals are measured in milligrams or micrograms; when combined, they will fit in a single tablet.

Fat, protein, and carbohydrate create other challenges that are more difficult to meet with supplements than are the vitamins and minerals. These nutrients require special dietary planning for several reasons:

- You probably require more protein than the average person because of malabsorption, increased loss, and increased basal metabolism (the least amount of energy required to maintain vital functions in an organism at complete rest).
- You must reduce fat from animal sources (bad fat) to help eliminate the cramps and diarrhea that come from poor absorption.
- You need to increase good fat, which you can easily do by adding olive and flax oils to your food.
- You need to get more calories from complex carbohydrates.

This strategy calls for attention to diet, and two steps are essential. The first is to avoid red meat and to eat high-protein, easily digestible foods, including fish, fowl, and eggs. The second is to get enough calories, which means getting more complex carbohydrates from foods that don't irritate the bowels, such as rice, potatoes, and pasta. Some high-fat foods, such as avocados, are excellent, and oils, such as flax and olive, can be generously added to food to help prevent flare-ups.

One way of meeting protein and calorie needs is to use a supplemental food. Products are available that can provide a nice tasty "shake" that's high in protein, with the correct amount of fat and moderate carbohydrates. Adding flax oil to the shake would increase its caloric delivery and help suppress inflammation. Managing inflammation with diet is discussed in more detail in Part II.

## Diarrhea and Nutrition

Diarrhea causes a loss of electrolytes, the salts (including sodium, chloride, and potassium) needed by your body to maintain correct fluid balance, nervous system function, and general health. Most of us get excess sodium and chloride, so the problem becomes one of not enough potassium. This is especially critical because potassium isn't easily taken as a supplement and must be obtained from the right vegetable foods. Avocados, ripe bananas, and orange juice are excellent potassium sources and should be frequently used by IBD patients.

Diarrhea also results from an inability of the swollen tissues to deal with excess bile acids, some of which are reabsorbed in the lower small intestine. Because the small intestine is impaired, the bile acids are passed into the large intestine, where they irritate and increase watery diarrhea. Excess bile acids cause the poor fat absorption that produces foul stools and watery diarrhea. The solution to this natural dilemma is to increase the soluble dietary fiber from foods such as oatmeal, which are rich in the right kind of fiber. When taken regularly, a refined soluble fiber supplement, such as Metamucil, can also help to firm up the stools by binding the bile acids. You just need to take enough; for example, a tablespoon in water at least four times daily stops the diarrhea and intestinal irritation.

## A Special Challenge: The K-Factor

The K-factor is the ratio of dietary potassium to sodium. We all require about 3,500 milligrams of potassium daily and can get along nicely on about 1,000 milligrams of sodium. However, we can tolerate up to 2,500 milligrams of sodium and even more if we get sufficient potassium. The K-factor ratio should always be at least 1 and preferably 3. This presents a special problem for people with IBD.

Potassium is easily eliminated in urine, and it is inadvertently lost in watery stools. The problem is that the only really good dietary sources of potassium are natural foods, especially fruits and vegetables. Most processed foods, particularly packaged foods, are loaded with sodium and seldom provide even half as much potassium. (Chapter Twenty-three covers this topic.) However, in this book you will often see reference to food as having a good K-factor, or as being a good source of potassium. My intention is to raise your awareness of your potassium need, which can't be overemphasized.

## Medication and Nutrition

Medication usually increases one or more nutritional requirements; no medication has been developed yet that decreases nutritional requirements! Most people have used aspirin and given baby aspirin to their children, but how many know that aspirin and its modern counterparts increase the need for vitamin C? How many people take some extra vitamin C and B with the aspirin? And keep in mind that aspirin is probably the simplest medication people use.

Medications used for IBD range from corticosteroids,

which increase the need for the B-complex of vitamins, to resins, which can reduce the absorption of important minerals and the water-soluble vitamins. Unfortunately, the nutritional effects of prescription drugs are seldom discussed by either your physician or your pharmacist.

There are several things the IBD sufferer can do. Make sure your diet meets the plan in this book and use the sensible nutritional supplements also discussed. Consult with your physician and, most of all, your pharmacist, who can give you detailed information on medication, and learn about the effects of your medication.

## Stress

IBD is stressful even if it is not stress related. Stress increases the nutritional requirements of normal people, so it follows that people with a chronic illness are more nutritionally challenged.

Diet can help to increase or moderate the effects of stress. When you eat food that's high in sugar, salt, caffeine, or saturated fat, you're stressing your body's ability to reestablish its normal balance. For example, excessive sugar first increases, then decreases, blood sugar; this can first make you a little sleepy and then anxious. A similar situation arises when you drink too much alcohol, which should generally be avoided by people with IBD.

Stress management with diet requires that you eat foods that do not contain empty calories from sugar or fat. Similarly, don't overwork your kidneys by eating foods with excessive sodium and not enough potassium, because it can interfere with your fluid balance.

## Caffeine

Anyone with IBD or another intestinal problem should select tea over coffee. Tea is much easier on the stomach, provides less caffeine with a milder stimulant effect, and doesn't require as much stomach acid production. In fact, tea actually speeds stomach emptying, which prevents an "acid" stomach.

Tea has been used for about 10,000 years and coffee for only about 3,000, but both beverages supply the same stimulant—caffeine. A typical cup of tea or a 12-ounce can of most colas provides about 40 milligrams of caffeine. A cup of coffee, in contrast, delivers from 100 to 150 milligrams of caffeine, depending on the brew. And the oils in coffee increase stomach acid output, so even decaffeinated coffee is not a solution for IBD patients.

Caffeine is an addictive alkaloid that stimulates the central nervous system. The lift from caffeine isn't generally harmful or as intense as other drugs, but it is addictive. When heavy coffee drinkers stop using coffee, they exhibit the same withdrawal symptoms—anxiety, irritability, paranoia, and even sickness—as hard drug users, although the symptoms aren't as intense.

Since caffeine stimulates the central nervous system, when the caffeine is gone, you feel more tired and seem to have less energy. Caffeine also increases your calcium requirement since coffee drinkers excrete more calcium than non-coffee drinkers. Milk or cream in coffee cannot possibly make up for this calcium loss, so you should rely on a calcium supplement. Or stop drinking coffee altogether!

## Serious Flare-ups

Serious flare-ups often call for a dramatic step—prescribing a complete predigested formula diet. Don't confuse these diets with the canned weight-loss products sold in the supermarket. "Predigested" doesn't mean the formula has been eaten or even artificially digested; it means all the nutritional requirements are in their basic form so your system isn't called upon to do anything except absorb nutrients. We call these formulas "low residue" because they are completely absorbed and have no fiber. The objective is to give your digestive system a complete rest. After a couple of weeks on these liquid products, when the flare-up has passed, you can slowly start eating foods, beginning with broth and working up slowly to easily digested carbohydrate-rich foods and moderately fat foods such as the white meat of fowl or any fish. Alternatively, you can continue with the medicinal liquid foods, but progress to those with complete protein and even some fiber.

Think of it as if you'd twisted your ankle badly. The doctor taped it and said, "Stay completely off it for a week; then you can slowly start walking carefully, perhaps with a cane at first, until it feels normal again." Your intestine is no different; it's got to rest, and the only way is to use predigested food.

## Enteral Nutrition

The next step beyond a predigested meal you drink is enteral nutrition, where a tube is inserted through your nose into your stomach. This tube is then attached to a solution of raw nutrients, amino acids, fatty acids, and appropriate sugars that are dripped slowly into the stomach. This "food" is easily absorbed and allows the intestine to rest. Enteral nutrition is often used with children and can bring IBD into remission. In recent years it has become the solution of choice to stop a flare-up and to avoid the use of steroids.

## TPN: Total Parenteral Nutrition

Use of total parenteral nutrition (TPN) started many years ago with people who were severely injured. These people didn't have enough small intestine left to get any nutrition. The only hope was to nourish them through a large vein. The process works and, thanks to dedicated researchers, has become a routine procedure.

Some people are alive today who haven't eaten in years. For instance, they may come home from a normal day's work and hook themselves up to a machine that pumps the elements of food into their bodies. By doing this, they don't just survive, they thrive! TPN is a high-tech answer to a problem that was once deadly—the ultimate marriage between nutrition and technology. Nutrients bypass the digestive system completely. People who must survive by this means can lead a relatively normal, productive, and abundant life.

TPN gives the small intestine a complete short-term rest. Think over the twisted ankle analogy. If the small intestine is in trouble, why not take the same approach? Give it a rest; let it heal. TPN is the answer physicians will choose for serious cases of IBD.

When on TPN, you're in the hands of a sophisticated team led by a physician, who is assisted by dietitians, nurses, medical technologists, and sociologists. They'll work together with the objective of restoring health to your digestive system and getting you back on real food.

## Steroid Use

For years an IBD flare-up was brought into remission by extensive steroid use, with all the unpleasant side effects that accompany those drugs. Health scientists have now compared steroid use to the three approaches just discussed. Their overwhelming conclusion: Avoid steroids if you can! Predigested food, enteral nutrition, and TPN are now the first choices in treatment.

The symptoms listed in Table 1.1 are often observed when people are marginally deficient in a particular nutrient. However, they are also associated with other more or less serious illnesses, complications of illness, or side effects of medication. If any of these symptoms persist, be sure your diet and dietary supplements are correct, and see your physician.

# CHAPTER 2

# Putting People's Experiences into Food

We'll discuss the basics of how nutrition and diet can be used to stop inflammation in Part II. But since you eat food, not nutrients, you've got to avoid foods that cause discomfort and select those that can help your illness subside. Experience and serious research teach that some foods are generally unacceptable for everyone with IBD, and some foods are universally acceptable and will help suppress inflammation. Everyone with IBD should choose foods from the latter category, learning to enjoy and use them to advantage. However, since we are all individuals, food that presents no problem for one person is not always okay for another.

## Flare-ups: Diarrhea

A flare-up usually involves serious pain and diarrhea (often bloody), which can be so devastating as to require hospitalization. As discussed in Chapter One, when this happens specialized feeding (with or without the use of steroids) is often used to speed remission. Remission is a period when there is no diarrhea, no blood, and normal (albeit possibly soft) stools. Improvement is defined as runny, but not watery, stools, with very little blood.

Surgery is the last resort for IBD patients. Carl, a psychologist, summarized his experience: "I couldn't conduct my professional practice because I would have to go to the bathroom so often. Patients would become irritated because it interrupted a train of thought, so I elected to have an ostomy. It has its difficulties, but I can now carry on a normal psychological counseling practice." Carl proves that even the last resort can be a doorway to a better life.

Surgery often involves removal of part of the bowel and is usually confined to a section of the large intestine. In many cases, the patient is left with a temporary or permanent *ostomy*. An ostomy is an opening in the abdomen, which allows stools to pass into a bag that you attach and remove yourself. The surgeon can often build an internal pouch that acts as a reservoir in which the waste collects; it is emptied into an appliance. Surgeons have other variations on these procedures and try to make life as normal as possible after surgery.

Many people have told me that surgery brings relief and at least allows them to live a normal life. Before that, any trip to the store or to visit a friend might end in a dash home because of painful cramps and diarrhea. People would even plan their vacations around their IBD, which often meant not having one. Even after surgery, however, many people continue to experience flare-ups. For them the specter of more surgery hangs heavy. Like everyone else with IBD, they must diligently practice prevention of flare-ups.

Foods can cause flare-ups and diarrhea. In some cases the flare-up follows immediately. As Betty put it, "I suspected beet juice as the culprit so I drank some. Within thirty minutes it was expelled in my watery stool!" She goes on to explain that for her, beet juice is like a diabolical poison. "I'd rather starve than drink it. I can't describe how devastating it is to me!" Actually, there's a slight misconception here; one cannot eat something and have it pass in thirty minutes. In this case beets are so irritating to Betty that they precipitate a violent reaction farther down the digestive tract, possibly including the passage of some blood.

Unlike Betty, a few people claim they can eat just about

anything and only have flare-ups twice a year—in spring and fall—no matter what they do. Their IBD flare-ups are triggered by something besides food, such as environmental changes. I suspect these could include sensitivity or even allergy to pollen; seasonal produce changes in the supermarket, which at first have a different or irritating component; and changes in barometric pressure. On the other hand, it is quite possible that seasonal shifts bring changes in normal daily patterns that are stressful even though they don't seem obvious.

## Foods That Cause Flare-ups and Diarrhea

As IBD continues to spread worldwide, more food-related studies are being conducted to settle on those foods that should always be avoided. Since this research has yielded consistent findings in many countries, it applies to all people. There is amazing consistency between the research and my anecdotal findings from more than 100 IBD patients or their parents whom I interviewed. Consequently, I have great confidence in the tabulations where I condense these findings (see Tables 2.1 and 2.2).

Scientific studies on food compare the food selections of IBD patients with those of people with the same demographics, such as ethnic background, age, weight, and socioeconomic status, who do not suffer from IBD. An analysis of this type deals with action, not thoughts or feelings; therefore, it applies to Hindus, Muslims, Christians, and Jews, and crosses skin color and other personal demographics. For example, if you find that the cultural foods are generally spicy (as in Thailand), but that IBD patients avoid spicy foods in both restaurants and grocery purchases, it's safe to say that spicy foods cause or aggravate flare-ups and diarrhea. Their actions, not the demographics, count.

The information I gained from interviews is anecdotal; in other words, the information given verbally to me is from experience and is not verified by taking samples of food actually eaten. Some clinical research involves giving people a capsule containing either a spice or a placebo with starch, and observing which causes a flare-up or aggravates diarrhea. Alternatively, people would be asked to eat specific foods in a predetermined sequence and researchers would observe who got sick and when. Some people would get sick enough to be hospitalized, possibly seriously enough to require TPN (total parenteral nutrition) or surgery. That type of research isn't justifiable, because we can learn the same things by simply interviewing many people and letting their experiences speak for themselves.

Table 2.1 lists foods that seem to consistently cause (or aggravate) flare-ups, discomfort, and diarrhea. These foods probably don't tell the entire story. Other patterns have emerged that make me suspect some food additives and methods of food preparation, which are summarized in Table 2.2. Approach these foods and cooking techniques with caution.

## Table 2.1

### Foods That Cause Flare-ups and Diarrhea

| Food | Examples |
| --- | --- |
| Spicy foods | Includes Mexican, some Italian food, and curry; spices such as cinnamon and ginger |
| Alcohol | All except a moderate amount of wine |
| Coffee | Some decaffeinated coffee requires testing |
| Chocolate | In any form, including candy and chocolate beverages |
| Raw vegetables | Corn, cabbage, beets, popcorn, etc. |
| Stringy meats | Stew meats, pot roast, Swiss steak, etc. |
| Nuts and seeds | Peanuts, almonds, sesame seeds; even seeds in rye bread cause trouble. (Many people identify nuts as a serious problem. It could be that the coarse pieces of nuts cause irritation. Try smooth peanut butter versus peanuts.) |

| Food | Examples |
| --- | --- |
| Fatty red meats | Includes beef, especially steak, and pork |
| Diet beverages | Includes carbonated and noncarbonated |
| Raw, unpeeled fruits | Apples, peaches, pears, grapes, etc. |
| Sugar | Cakes, icing, soft drinks |
| Food additives | Monosodium glutamate (MSG), possibly saccharine |
| Processed meats | Sausage, cold cuts such as bologna, salami, etc., frankfurters |
| Dairy products | Whole milk, ice cream, some cheese; some low-fat or nonfat milk is all right, especially on softened cereal |
| Desserts | Ice cream, cream pie, cheese cake, chocolate |
| Shellfish | Clams, oysters, mussels; crustaceans such as shrimp, lobster, crabs |

## Table 2.2

### Food Preparation Methods That Cause Flare-ups

| | |
| --- | --- |
| Pickling | Pickled vegetables, such as sauerkraut, pickles, relishes |
| Gravy | Meats that are well tolerated, such as chicken and turkey, can cause flare-ups when gravy is added |
| Uncooked vegetables | Vegetables cooked to softness are all right. |
| Crispy vegetables | Vegetables steamed, but still crispy to the bite. |
| Frying | Foods that are well tolerated, such as fish, will cause flare-ups if they're deep-fat or pan-fried in oil |
| Charcoal broiling to charred | Any charred meat or fish causes trouble |

Foods flavored with MSG (monosodium glutamate) were a problem for most people. Apples caused discomfort in some people, so they stopped eating them. Others peeled the apples and removed the core and found they were just fine. The same approach worked for peaches, pears, grapes, and plums. Baking apples or poaching pears, which breaks up the fiber matrix, made them fine for some people, as long as the skin was removed.

## Foods That Didn't Cause Flare-ups

The foods listed below are the ones that *most* people with IBD could usually eat with no discomfort. I emphasize *most* because not everyone could eat all of them. Some people ate almost any food in moderation, but were very careful with preparation. This listing proves that there are many foods to choose from, enough to make eating varied and pleasurable. I've listed them by category and noted any pertinent facts about preparation.

*Cereal:* Oatmeal, Cream of Wheat, cornflakes, bran flakes, Malt-O-Meal, Special K, Product 19, and Cheerios. Avoid hard-fiber ("fiber matrix") wheat cereals such as All-Bran. It is best to avoid milk and use soy or rice "milk" in its place.

*Dairy products:* Lactaid milk, low-fat and nonfat (skim) milk, yogurt, aged cheese, cottage and soft cheese, and soy beverages.

*Eggs:* People who ate eggs emphasized poached, soft boiled, and hard boiled. Not a single respondent could eat fried eggs, which is consistent with intolerance of all fried foods. Eggs are universally one of, if not *the* best, most economical source of protein available, so it's worthwhile to try various cooking methods.

*Meat:* Some people could eat beef, lean ham, carefully trimmed pork, trimmed lamb, and veal. If you can, I suggest you do so only once monthly. Emphasis must always be on "lean" and "trimmed." Clinical research has turned up a possible predisposing effect of beef and other red meat on IBD. Reducing animal fat is essential to stopping inflammation, so learn to get along without red meats.

*Fish:* Fish was universally accepted. Eating fish, especially cold-water fish with dark skin, is important to prevent inflammation. The oils in fish are essential and have a proven therapeutic benefit. Emphasize fish that swim, called finfish, which include tuna, swordfish, salmon, halibut, and flounder. Preparation includes broiling, poaching, and baking. *Do not fry!*

*Shellfish:* Scallops are all right if broiled or poached. Studiously avoid all other shellfish, such as clams and oysters, and crustaceans, including lobster and crab.

*Poultry:* Everyone who responded could eat white breast meat of poultry, but the skin must be removed and the meat cannot be fried or breaded. Always avoid dark poultry meat.

*Vegetables:* I divided the wide variety of vegetables into categories most people are familiar with.

*Potatoes:* Always eat potatoes (baked, boiled, or mashed) without the skin. Sweet potatoes and yams are fine if well cooked and peeled.

*Vegetables with skin:* Remove the skin from carrots, squash, tomatoes, cucumbers, celery, jicama, and others. These vegetables should be cooked (steamed, boiled, or baked) until they are definitely soft enough to mash with a fork. Cooking to softness flies in the face of what most people do, but most people don't have IBD. While you lose some of the vitamins, you gain the essential fiber, minerals, and most antioxidants. You'll have to take vitamin supplements in any event.

*Vegetables without skin:* Broccoli, cauliflower, brussels sprouts, asparagus, all string beans, and peas must be cooked well by boiling or steaming until soft. Do not eat crisp vegetables.

*Beans:* Some beans can simply be boiled with two or three water changes; these include limas, navy beans, and lentils. Other beans, such as black, pinto, kidney, red, and garbanzos, must be boiled with two or three water changes so they can be mashed or easily pureed in a blender. Most people can eat canned baked beans provided they have no pork or animal fat (lard).

*Leafy vegetables:* Lettuce is fine for everyone. Spinach is all right for most people when boiled to softness. Cabbage, if boiled to softness, is acceptable to some people, but others insist they must avoid it at all costs; therefore, I would put it on a "dangerous" or "caution" list.

*Fruit:* Emphasis should be placed on peeling. It seems that most fruits, including apples, pears, peaches, and avocados, are acceptable if they've been peeled; for citrus fruits, the white fibrous material must be removed with the peel. Avocados provide excellent oils and are one of the richest sources of potassium, two serious needs for people with IBD. In my studies, I didn't encounter anyone who couldn't eat ripe avocados, well-ripened bananas (not green), apricots (if fully ripe and peeled), plums (if fully ripe and peeled), strawberries, kiwifruit, canned fruits (canning softens the fiber matrix), oranges, and grapefruit. (Remember to carefully avoid and remove the fibrous sections of grapefruit, oranges, tangerines, lemons, and limes.)

*Grains:* Boiled white and brown rice and pasta. Breads and rolls without seeds, including white, rye, wheat, five-grain, French, and Italian. Absolutely *no seeds of any type*— sesame, poppy, rye, etc.

*Processed foods:* Some processed foods are excellent: canned fruits, apple sauce, canned vegetables, baked beans.

*Beverages:* Most people could tolerate fruit juices, such as orange, grapefruit, cranberry, and apple, and vegetable juices, such as tomato and V-8 juice.

Modern technology has given us calcium-fortified frozen orange juice, which provides 300 milligrams of calcium per serving. Freezing does not detract from the nutrient delivery of orange or other juices; in fact, it breaks down the fiber matrix. Orange juice is an excellent source of potassium (480 milligrams) and vitamin C, so it's an ideal beverage for active people, and anytime you have had diarrhea.

Hot tea is fine and iced is all right; caffeine-free cola and other carbonated beverages, such as ginger ale and 7UP, not artificially sweetened; mineral water, distilled water, and reverse-osmosis purified water; limeade; herb tea; and soy beverages.

## What I've Learned from the Eating Patterns

By trial and error, guidance from physicians, and talking to other people, IBD sufferers can learn what's okay for them. A careful food diary is an excellent asset to discover what works for you, but there are some basics that apply to everyone.

Small portions and more frequent meals seem to be a universally acceptable pattern. Surprisingly, this is a much healthier way for everyone to eat. If portions and meals are kept small, a wider variety of food is acceptable. That's logical because the intestine doesn't need to deal with a large quantity of any single material, and a small meal is more likely to be well chewed. There are portion thresholds for most foods that cause or aggravate flare-ups. For example, you might be able to tolerate half an orange, or a small serving of beans, but an entire orange or a full serving of beans could set you off. In any case, always remember to *chew food thoroughly.*

It's often good to puree a tomato sauce for pasta after it has been prepared. Some fruits, such as bananas and even peeled apples, can be blended with orange juice for a smoothie. Go easy on ice since cold beverages and cold food cause trouble for many people. Gravy and rich sauces always spell trouble.

Fiber is helpful; oatmeal, bananas, and most peeled fruit are excellent. However, a fiber matrix, such as a fruit peel or a hard bean coat, especially wheat bran, is out. Cereals with soluble fiber, such as oatmeal, are ideal, and fiber supplements such as Metamucil are beneficial, if not therapeutic.

Most of the people with IBD I interviewed avoided fried foods and large portions of fatty meats, which highlights their inability to tolerate these foods. Fat is often associated with tough membranes, which could irritate the intestinal wall in the same way an apple peel does. Nonetheless, animal or saturated fat itself is definitely a problem. The white meat, rather than dark, of poultry and fish were generally well tolerated by people I interviewed. Overall, a diet low in animal fat is best for people with IBD. In Part II, I will explain how it reduces inflammation and tissue damage. These observations made me curious about food as a therapeutic aid, so I asked another question: "Are there any foods that stop flare-ups or diarrhea?"

## Foods That Help Stop Flare-ups and Diarrhea

EILEEN: *"If there was a single food to stop the flare-ups I'd be at the grocery store and not the hospital."*

Eileen was writing to me from her hospital bed!

There are supplemental foods that can help rest the bowels while giving complete nutrition. Criticare HN by Bristol-Myers and Vital HN by Ross Laboratories come as close to complete digestive rest as possible with excellent nutritional support. When IBD patients don't eat, they risk serious illness due to loss of electrolytes and other nutrients. Criticare and Vital prevent nutrient deficiency and bring them through the storm while resting the digestive system.

Soft soluble fiber supplements such as Metamucil help stop diarrhea and bind the stools. I suggest you use six servings as described on the label, appropriately spaced, on a daily basis as a standard supplement. Creamy oatmeal made by slow cooking and Cream of Wheat seem to help most people with IBD. Some patients eat ripe bananas, mashed potatoes, or well-cooked rice, remedies based on personal experimentation.

An old folk remedy for diarrhea recommends eating an apple (peeled, of course), banana, and cottage cheese. The apple and banana supply soluble fiber, and calcium from the cheese adds more binding capacity. The combination also helps restore the electrolyte balance. The original research done on fiber by Neil Painter, an English physician, included people with the "diarrhea disease" (chronic diarrhea, even though it had not been officially diagnosed as IBD). Adding fiber to their food stopped the diarrhea and normalized their bowels.

Most average people, and IBD patients in particular, don't get nearly enough fiber. This observation is confirmed by research done on people with IBD in Europe, the United States, and Asia. Those who get the most fiber eat oatmeal, fruit, potatoes, brown rice, and vegetables without skin.

The fiber in bran or whole-grain cereals is retained from the original plant cell wall and could be very irritating for an inflamed bowel. Thus, people with IBD should be careful when selecting cereals. In Chapter Six we'll review the cereals that provide the best dietary fiber.

## Vitamin and Mineral Supplements

Many people use food supplements prescribed by doctors. People who are missing the lower part of the small intestine (largely as a result of surgery), require $B_{12}$ injections. Most supplements (see Chapter Seven) provide a good balance of vitamins and minerals, but they cannot compensate for potassium, fiber, or protein, which are covered in other chapters.

Hanna, a Crohn's patient, put it very clearly:

*"I started taking supplements in 1983. I've progressively improved since then. Through good nutrition, I have built up my body to a point where my Crohn's disease is not as severe as in the past. I have small flare-ups now as compared to chronic, life-threatening episodes where I would be hospitalized. My health improved so much that I didn't think twice about becoming pregnant in 1985."*

I was surprised at how sensibly people selected their food supplements. In addition to a multivitamin-multimineral supplement, people selected supplements to meet their individual needs. They used calcium, calcium and magnesium, iron, zinc, B-complex, vitamin C, vitamin E, and beta carotene.

The people who use supplements seem to have a more positive attitude and require less medication.

## Medications

The number of medications used by IBD patients can be overwhelming. Some people take as many as twenty tablets and capsules daily, not counting vitamin supplements. The following list gives you an idea of the variety and scope. Not all of them are used for IBD; the list contains medications for asthma, anxiety, insomnia, motion sickness, and high blood pressure, as well as antipsychotics and one or two potassium supplements. Potassium supplements aren't recommended since they often irritate the intestine. It's easier (and more tasty) to get potassium from your food.

| | |
|---|---|
| ACTH | Lomotil |
| Azulfidine (sulfasalazine) | Medrol |
| Bentyl | Norpace |
| Bumex | Parafon Forte |
| Capoten | Prednisone |
| Cardizem | Premarin |
| Chlorthalidone | Provera |
| Compazine | Questran |
| Corgard | Restoril |
| Darvocet | Seldane |
| Desyrel | Serax |
| Dyazide | Tagamet |
| Elavil | Theo-Dur |
| Flagyl | Thyroid medication |
| Halcion | Tranxene |
| Imodium | Xanax |
| K-Lyte | Zyloprim |
| Lasix | |

## Supplements and Medication

Most medication increases the need for nutrients, and some medication prevents the absorption of nutrients. What's a person to do? Take a complete, balanced food supplement (see Chapter Seven) daily, together with specific vitamins and minerals that are especially vulnerable, including folic acid, calcium, magnesium, zinc, and vitamin C.

# CHAPTER 3

# *Food and Lifestyle Diary*

A food and lifestyle diary is the simplest and most direct way to find out what foods and food preparation methods cause flare-ups. For a very small time investment, you can improve your health, learn more about yourself, and become a solid partner with your doctor. It is "self-health management" at its best.

In Chapter Two we reviewed foods and cooking methods that cause and prevent flare-ups, and we also discussed the clinical research. Clinicians noted an inconsistency in how foods affected people with IBD. Each person seemed to be sensitive to certain foods that others could eat regularly. Unfortunately, in a clinical setting there is no way for scientists to evaluate cooking methods, or even to be aware of every ingredient used. Consequently, when a particular food causes one person trouble but doesn't bother another, variables such as cooking techniques, an unmentioned ingredient, and how well the person chews food may explain the discrepancy. Each adult with IBD, or the parent of a child with the disease, should take charge of diet by keeping a food diary.

## Self-health Management

At a lecture, I convinced an audience member named Phyllis to keep a food diary. She knew she developed canker-like sores inside her mouth three to five days before a flare-up. Phyllis started keeping a food diary and noted that the canker sores appeared two to three days after eating tangerines. She told her doctor about these sores, and he prescribed medication for them, which made the flare-up milder. However, it was actually the tangerines that Phyllis would eat several times a day when they were in season that were causing the sores.

Phyllis learned she could cause flare-ups by eating several tangerines or mandarin oranges. By trial and error she found that the canned fruit equivalent didn't cause any problem, and that she could tolerate about half of a fresh tangerine.

Isn't Phyllis's story informative and simple? All she did was keep track of what she ate and drank, how it was prepared, how much she ate, why she ate it, and how she felt at the time.

By using this simple notebook, Phyllis learned how to control her IBD and enjoy a favorite food. She can even explain why canned tangerines were okay.

In a subsequent test she realized that she often peeled the tangerines quickly, leaving the white fibrous material (membrane) on them. She learned that if she carefully removed the membrane she could usually eat a whole tangerine with no consequences. In canned tangerines, the membrane is removed by processing. Tangerines are also moderately cooked in the canning process, which helps to break down the fiber matrix.

The diary concept doesn't stop with food. When you record how you feel emotionally—what caused your stress, anger, or fear, or simply upset you—patterns sometimes emerge that will allow you to avoid sources of stress.

For example, Russ noticed his flare-ups coincided with visits to his in-laws. At first he blamed his mother-in-law's cooking, so on the next trip, his wife took over in the kitchen. A flare-up started about a half an hour into the ride home.

"Could it be an emotional problem?" I asked.

Russ observed that his father-in-law, a very successful engineer and manager, "knew everything" and would counter most of the comments he offered in conversations. Consequently, Russ kept his feelings to himself (not uncommon for Crohn's patients) and let them ferment. I call this *implosion.*

If Russ had kept a diary, he would have recognized that his mother-in-law's cooking was not the problem. He could have reasoned from his notes that he often left his in-laws' home "tied in knots."

To address the issue of stress, Russ cut their future family visits short, avoided conversations about deep subjects, and focused on his children or on his wife's interests. Russ also took extra fiber supplements, which we'll discuss in Chapter Sixteen. The result was less controversy, and the "in-law" flare-ups disappeared.

## Details of the Diary

There's no correct way to keep a food diary, but after working with several groups of people who have arthritis, asthma, and other inflammatory illnesses, I can tell you what works best for them. It's easy.

Start by purchasing a spiral notebook, one that is at least 9½ inches by 6 inches. I prefer the standard 8½ inches by 11 inches, but the smaller one fits in pocketbooks, so it's more convenient. People who use a briefcase can buy the larger size. Whatever works is okay.

Date each page and start by noting how you feel when you get up. Morning is an important time, because during the day, in the middle of daily activities, we often suppress feelings of discomfort. In addition, when you're active, your brain produces chemicals called *endorphins.* Endorphins, also called "natural opiates," have a mood-lifting effect, so you're likely not to recognize mild discomfort when your brain is producing them. In the morning, the previous day's endorphins are gone, so you start to feel your discomforts again.

Write down what you eat during the day. Be as specific as possible. If you started the day with a bowl of cereal, note the type: Was it oatmeal, corn bran, or some other kind? Did you use skim milk, 1 percent milk, soy beverage, or Lactaid? How much? Did you add sugar? Be as specific as possible about food. For example, don't just list "potatoes"; write down if they were white, red, or sweet, how they were prepared, and if the skin was removed.

It's essential that you record everything: meals, snacks, and beverages. There's no way to be certain ahead of time what will cause or aggravate a flare-up. In addition, a flare-up can be a reaction to a combination of foods, or the interaction between food and medication (also record when and what medications you take). You're looking for anything that can cause trouble, and once you've found it, you're in control! There's an alternative to any food, food combination, or cooking method.

Food preparation is critical. Note how the food was cooked, what condiments were used, and other subtleties. For example, did you peel the apple before or after you baked it? Were the vegetables crisp or cooked until soft? (Soft is always better.) Any characteristic of the food is important, including whether it was baked, boiled, or grilled. (Fried is always unacceptable!) Was the orange juice you drank at breakfast fresh, frozen reconstituted, or pasteurized bottled? Was it with or without pulp?

Serving size or the amount eaten is second in importance after the food itself. Experience will help you to estimate correct portions. Some things are easy to measure, such as fruits or vegetables. But how much cereal did you eat? You simply poured it from the box to the bowl. How much milk or soy beverage did you use? Learn to use a measuring cup to get a feeling for what a half or a third of a cup of cereal looks like. Do the same thing with spaghetti, rice, and other commonly used foods. We seldom measure our food, but it can pay big dividends when we do.

If you're using food supplements, a fiber supplement, or a supplemental food, it's important to note the brand and how much you take. Choose fiber supplements with appropriate bowel movements in mind. If you've chosen correctly, and are using enough, the frequency and consistency of your bowel movements will be your guide. Stool frequency, size, color, odor, and even time after eating are important factors. Ideally, you should strive to have one bowel movement in twenty-four hours.

Where you eat is also an important environmental factor, as Russ's story illustrates.

Next, grade your food selection. How did you do nutritionally? Did you get everything you needed from your food? Did your supplements provide general nutrition and make up for specific shortfalls, such as calcium? If you took fiber supplements, were they enough? You're trying to get maximum benefit from food and should strive to get it right.

At the end of the day, critique your choices. First note how you feel. Then identify any unusual physiological events, either positive or negative. For example, if you had seven watery stools, it's important to note that. And if you had one with good consistency, it's also important to write it down, because it means you're doing something right. A major change will help you identify a problem food. Next, evaluate the emotional events of the day. If things were average, that's okay. But if there was some unusual stress or emotional upheaval, identify it, analyze it, and remember it, because if you wake up the next day feeling sick, it could be the cause. More important, the emotional upset could contribute to your flare-up as much as the food.

Finally, write down any body changes. Recognize that an intestinal upheaval is often preceded by sores, an aching joint, a headache, a rash, or some other nonintestinal manifestation. These are of immense importance, because once you learn to identify them, you will learn what foods or preparation methods to avoid. If you can anticipate a flare-up, you can inform your doctor so he or she can prescribe medication to prevent or lessen its effects.

## When a Food Causes a Reaction

Let's say you've used a food diary and some food you've eaten causes a reaction. Should you eliminate it? Not until you've tested it a couple of times under different circumstances. Suppose you eat brussels sprouts with foods you know are safe, and you end up with a long bout of diarrhea or a case of abdominal cramps. Let things return to normal, then try the same food again, using a small amount with a food you know is bland, like mashed potatoes. If you get a reaction, it's probably the brussels sprouts, but it's probably worth one more try with a similar small amount and another safe food. A third reaction means you should put it on your "avoid" list.

Try these foods again in a year or two to see if they're still a problem. Food sensitivities have a way of slowly changing, so you must keep testing.

## Food Diary Versus Elimination Diet

Some doctors use an *elimination diet*. This is a program in which certain foods are added and some eliminated. It's excellent for identifying food groups and even specific foods that cause trouble. For example, suppose you have chronic diarrhea. You eliminate all wheat-containing foods and the diarrhea clears up. You could be sensitive to wheat; in fact, you might even be unable to tolerate a wheat protein called gluten. But even an elimination diet won't replace a food and lifestyle diary.

An elimination diet sounds like an easy procedure, but it is very sophisticated and requires professional supervision. There are several critical variations, such as eliminating one group before another. Even if your doctor prescribes an elimination diet, maintain your diary to make the entire process more effective. You'll be able to spot things that the elimination diet is likely to miss. For example, do canker sores or red lumps precede an intestinal flare-up? If they do, you'll know it much sooner with the diary than the diet. So use both.

## Sensitivity Subtleties

As I've noted, food sensitivities aren't allergies. For example, suppose you eat some zucchini bread you've been given and notice a canker sore two days later. Worse yet, suppose one piece doesn't trigger the sore, and you have to eat it on three consecutive days in order to get a reaction. It will be hard enough to sort out this subtle relationship with a food diary, and impossible without one. Once you've traced it to the bread, you then must determine if it's the zucchini or something else in the bread.

For a previous book, I asked people to test foods for arthritis flare-ups. Two women made the scope of their reactions very clear. Here is a summary of their stories:

BETTY: *"I can eat an egg one day, an egg the second day, but if I eat an egg the third day, I can't get out of bed on the fourth day."*

Betty needed perseverance to learn that about herself. She had to keep a food diary. Norma's story is a little different; she had stopped eating all organ meats as my program had instructed.

NORMA: *"My daughter made the honor society and I attended the parents' dinner reception. They had chicken liver hors d'oeuvres; without thinking I ate mine completely. I was so sick the next day I couldn't walk. I forgot how far I had come."*

Norma had forgotten how sensitive she is to meats. New habits had taken over. She had taken her newfound health for granted; the dinner reception flare-up snapped her back to reality.

I don't think ten experts would agree on how to describe each woman's different reaction to food. Some would say: "It's in her head!" In fact, I wrote a book with exactly that title because it was not in either woman's head. Some would say: "Allergy!" I might agree in Norma's case, but not Betty's. If each has allergies, they're as different as night and day. Some would say: "Food sensitivity!" I'd certainly agree in Betty's case, but would have doubts in Norma's. It's a complex problem, and labeling it doesn't make it go away.

Only two points are clear: Betty can eat eggs if she's careful, and Norma can't eat chicken livers. Neither one needs to experiment with her sensitivity any further. That's what I call self-health management.

# CHAPTER 4

# Milk and Lactose Intolerance

More than 80 percent of all adults can't drink over 6 ounces of milk without developing abdominal cramps or diarrhea or a bloated feeling, and sometimes all three. These are symptoms of lactose intolerance. Lactose is milk sugar, and it's the main carbohydrate in human milk and cow's milk. By age 6, many people, especially blacks, Asians, and most ethnic Mediterranean people, lose their ability to digest lactose. Most Northern European Caucasians retain their ability to digest lactose as long as they continue drinking milk. People with IBD are usually, if not always, lactose intolerant.

## Lois's Story

Lois is an attractive young woman with Crohn's disease. On a speaking tour for which she was hostess, I noticed that she usually included a glass of milk at every meal. After drinking the milk and before the meal was finished, Lois took at least one trip to the lavatory.

I suggested that Lois not drink milk for at least one week. The trips to the lavatory during meals stopped. I asked her if she noticed the difference. "Yes," she said, "I never realized that milk was doing that." "Did you ever get cramps or feel nauseated?" I asked. "No," she replied, "only the runs."

Lois is lactose intolerant, but she doesn't get cramps, nausea, or bloating—just diarrhea. Her case is another example of why anyone with a chronic illness, especially an intestinal disorder, should keep an accurate food diary. If Lois had taken an aggressive attitude toward her own health, she would have related milk to diarrhea and searched for an alternative. Instead, she subconsciously adapted to the diarrhea that followed the milk.

## Cheese and Yogurt

Fermented dairy products solve two problems very nicely. In fermentation, most lactose breaks down or other sugars are produced and the protein and calcium of milk remain. That's why most cultures that can't drink milk have traditionally used cheese and yogurt. They preserve milk's excellent nutrition indefinitely, and they can be tolerated by lactose-intolerant people. Most IBD patients can eat yogurt and some cheese with no side effects. Nevertheless, most cheese has a lot of sodium and animal fat; therefore, it should be used in moderation (see Part II).

## Technology Rescues Milk

Why not add the enzyme lactase to milk and break down the lactose to glucose and galactose, which are simple sugars needing no further digestion? If you're lactose intolerant, that's exactly what you can do.

*Lactaid brand milk,* sold in most supermarkets, is treated with the enzyme lactase, which predigests the lactose. More than 70 percent of the lactose has been eliminated, and the remainder is about what you'd get in cheese. For example, 8 ounces of milk contains about 6 grams of lactose, so less than 1.8 grams of lactose remains in Lactaid milk. That is not enough to cause a reaction in even the most sensitive people. Even if the remaining lactose is a problem, you can totally eliminate it by adding *Lactaid Drops.* Lactaid Drops is a liquid preparation of the enzyme lactase that is readily available in drugstores. When added to milk, these drops eliminate more than 99 percent of all lactose. So, if you're lactose intolerant and use Lactaid Drops according to the directions, you can drink milk! There will be no symptoms of lactose intolerance, and you'll get all the nutrition that milk can provide.

There's still one more option. *Lactaid Caplets* (also found in drugstores) is a preparation of the enzyme lactase designed to work in the human stomach and small intestine. You simply take from one-half to three caplets at the beginning of a meal, depending on the amount of milk you intend to drink. That's all there is to solving lactose intolerance.

## Sugar Alcohol Intolerance

Sugar alcohols, especially sorbitol and maltitol, are used in some confection products and liquid-vitamin preparations. These sweet alcohols occur naturally in very small amounts in most fruit and are easily metabolized. However, large amounts of them can cause discomfort and illness in some people.

In this case, there's no alternative enzyme preparation similar to Lactaid. Therefore, read the ingredient list on any confection products and if sorbitol, maltitol, or xylitol appears on the ingredient list, use the product very cautiously. Don't tempt illness.

## Milk Allergy

Some people are actually allergic or sensitive to milk. While these milk allergies are mostly anecdotal, more and more pediatricians and physicians are recommending the use of milk alternatives. They cite symptoms such as excessive mucus congestion, and, in children, ear problems. When so many pediatricians take a position, I pay attention. It is one more reason why you may want to test an alternative to milk.

## Milk Alternatives

Soy or rice beverages (and, where it's available, almond milk) offer yet another solution to milk intolerance. These products have no lactose and can generally be tolerated by all people with intestinal disorders. The added advantage is that they deliver some extraordinary plant components that have proven anticancer properties.

Our need for calcium and protein are two good reasons why fermented milk products, such as cheese and yogurt, have been used for centuries. Protein insufficiency is no longer a problem in our society, since other sources are abundant, and calcium can be obtained in supplements and in fortified orange juice, which also provides an abundance of potassium (a problem nutrient for people with intestinal disorders).

# CHAPTER 5

# Fiber: The Forgotten Nutrient

I have noticed that many of you with IBD tend to eliminate fibrous foods from your diets, so you are inclined to eat highly processed foods that increase sugar and salt consumption disproportionately. But you need all the health benefits that fiber and fibrous foods provide, which are very positive, almost therapeutic.

## Fiber Matrix Problems

We briefly touched on fiber matrix in Chapter Two, so you know it as the peel on fruits, the coating of a seed, the tough outer skin on asparagus, and, at the extreme end, the woody stems of trees. I don't want you to eat trees, but I want you to understand that even the fiber matrix in trees can be turned to mush to make paper. Most of the time you can eliminate the matrix: peel the apple, remove the potato skin, or cook asparagus, string beans, spinach, and other vegetables until they're soft enough to mash with a fork. It's currently in vogue to eat crisp vegetables, which is obviously not good for people with IBD. But don't dismay; being different is what life is all about. Be sure to read Chapter Sixteen for a more thorough foundation on dietary fiber.

## Softening the Matrix

Insoluble fiber must be softened for people with IBD. This means that vegetables need to be cooked until their consistency is very soft. Although many people like vegetables such as broccoli crisp and crunchy—and some nutritionists advocate preparing them that way to capture every last nutrient—this quick-cooking method isn't for people with IBD. For them, it's important to boil, steam, or bake broccoli until the stems are soft. This applies to all vegetables that most people like to eat crunchy, including asparagus, carrots, zucchini, and squash. Don't worry about losing the vitamins; you can always take an extra vitamin pill! Some vegetables that can cause problems when eaten raw, such as peppers, should also be cooked. Microwaving is an acceptable cooking method; remember to cook all vegetables until soft.

When you cook vegetables until soft, especially stemmed vegetables like asparagus and broccoli, you are breaking down the fiber matrix but are still getting all the nourishment of fiber. After reading more than 100 IBD food questionnaires and interviewing as many IBD patients, I'm convinced that the fiber matrix, if not fully softened, irritates an inflamed bowel and is the reason why fresh vegetables cause flare-ups. The culprit isn't vegetables, it's the preparation, and that can be controlled.

## Canned Vegetables in Moderation

The canning process involves placing the vegetables in a water bath in which the temperature is elevated almost to boiling. Canners call this process "retorting" and a housewife would call it "pressure-cooking," but the result is the same: it breaks down the fiber matrix. Although the softness of commercially canned vegetables is good for people with IBD, the excess salt used in canning is a serious concern. So, at least remove the fluid in the can before cooking and use water to reduce the salt content. Commercially canned vegetables have a very poor K-factor—ratio of potassium to sodium—

(see Chapter Twenty-three); therefore, don't depend on them too much.

## Pressure-cooking Is Best

Pressure-cooking (or home canning) breaks the fiber matrix most efficiently. Instead of adding salt, use some olive oil for flavor and good health. An advantage of pressure-cooking is that it softens the vegetables, and you can save the liquid for soup and other recipes because it has excellent nutritional value and flavor. Pressure-cooking works on just about any vegetable you can name, even cabbages.

## Peel Fruits

If there's an insurmountable fiber matrix in the vegetable kingdom, it's the skin of fruits such as apples, pears, peaches, kiwifruit, berries, tomatoes, grapes, and plums. Always peel fruits! One clear correlation scientists have found is that grapes cause flare-ups, and my questionnaire proved it as well. How many people peel grapes? How many people eat seeded grapes without swallowing an occasional seed? Grapes are not for IBD patients.

## Ripe Fruit

Most fruits, including avocados, pears, plums, peaches, apricots, and melons, are shipped to the store when they're firm, even unripe. Shipping unripe fruits is good for the store, because firm fruits last longer; however, it's not good for the person with IBD.

While most people with IBD can eat ripe bananas, many say they get a flare-up or diarrhea from eating a slightly green banana. A greenish banana is ripe, but much of its fiber matrix is still intact. Let the banana ripen to yellow with brown spots before eating; it provides excellent soluble fiber.

Ripen all fruits before eating them. This may take days or even a week; some fruits, such as melons, need to be placed in a brown paper bag to ripen more quickly. An excellent way to tell that a pear is fully ripe is when it can be eaten with a spoon. Slice it in half, scoop out the seeds and core, and enjoy.

## Canned Fruits

Canned fruits are an excellent compromise for people with IBD. Canned fruits have been peeled and cooked, and their fiber matrix has generally been broken down. Fruits canned in natural juice are available and should be your fruits of choice. However, if you must buy the variety canned in sugar syrup, drain the fruit before eating it so you aren't getting all that sugar. Canned fruits are peeled before canning, often even grapes and tomatoes. Canned citrus fruits come in "sections" with the white matrix removed, making them very convenient and safe to eat. And as we discussed earlier, most people who keep a food diary conclude that the white fibrous material causes them trouble.

## Cereals

Cooked oatmeal is an ideal cereal, because oats are primarily a soluble fiber cereal. If oatmeal is started in cold water, cooked slowly, and allowed to become creamy, it is almost therapeutic for IBD. Many people have said that oatmeal slows down diarrhea and calms a flare-up. This is exactly what the scientific findings on dietary fiber indicate. Similar comments have been applied to cooked brown rice and Cream of Wheat. These cereals have two similarities: they are all good sources of soluble fiber and the fact that they are cooked means the fiber matrix has been broken down.

Flax cereal sold in some supermarkets and health food stores has an added advantage: it provides good soft fiber and also includes some flax oil, which by itself tends to help IBD and reduce heart disease. In Chapter Fourteen you will learn that flax oil is an omega-3 oil that, when appropriately used, can help to suppress inflammation.

In contrast to hot cereals, high-fiber cereals, such as All-Bran, All-Bran with Added Fiber, and similar high–wheat bran cereals, provide a large amount of hard, insoluble wheat fiber with a partially intact fiber matrix. Some studies and anecdotal reports indicate that high-fiber cereals like these can actually irritate the intestinal lining. And since these cereals usually aren't cooked, the matrix isn't broken down. Alternatives are the lower-fiber flaked cereals, such as Bran Flakes, Oat Flakes, Puffed Wheat, and Cheerios. While I don't have many reports on corn bran, I believe it is fine for IBD since its fiber is soft, and it softens even more in milk or soy beverage.

## Fiber Supplements

Metamucil is the standard against which I measure all fiber supplements. In my opinion, it is safe and consistent. Select the version that is not artificially sweetened; it comes unflavored and orange flavor, either of which is fine. You can take as much Metamucil as you desire. Indeed, it is probably acceptable to take up to six or more tablespoon servings daily. I should point out that it has been clinically tested and doesn't cause flare-ups.

Drugstores have a wide selection of fiber supplements besides Metamucil. Most of them are made from psyllium seeds, which are mostly *mucilage,* a type of fiber. They don't contain the seed matrix, are gentle, and also work well. On recommendation of a physician, they are often used to slow down and stop diarrhea and even quell an IBD flare-up. Make sure the one you choose is only a fiber supplement and does not contain any laxative.

A word of caution: Some fiber products actually contain senna leaf, an intestinal stimulant. Not only is senna a poor source of dietary fiber, but it can wreak havoc in IBD sufferers. Read the ingredients list carefully and avoid anything with senna or another "natural herbal laxative." Just because something is natural, it doesn't mean it's "safe."

Some health food stores sell plant gums, the most common being guar gum, which is also the most effective fiber for slowing diarrhea. However, guar gum should be used carefully because too much will "gum" the works, actually causing a blockage. I'll discuss this further in Chapter Sixteen, but for now my advice is to start slowly, follow directions carefully, and drink lots of water when consuming any fiber, especially gums and mucilages.

# CHAPTER 6

# Do's, Don'ts, and Cautions of Food Selection

You can reduce your flare-ups and help keep your IBD in remission with the foods you select. This chapter has only that purpose in mind. When I explain inflammation and its dietary management in Part II, you will understand why some foods are excluded and others emphasized.

I call foods you should be able to eat "Do's," foods you should never eat again "Don'ts," and foods you should experiment with "Cautions." Use caution foods carefully, because the experiences of many people indicate they can cause trouble.

## Read Labels

Modern supermarkets have up to 18,000 different food selections! Every year at least 1,800 items are either replaced by completely new products or altered by some new ingredients or processes, and that doesn't include produce, which also changes. Add to that number regional variations, because many supermarkets have their own bakeries and purchase local produce, as well as local meat and fish. Some supermarkets also cater to local ethnic populations, such as Spanish, Asian, and Middle Eastern. Therefore, while I can't tell you what packaged foods to purchase, I can show you how to read labels.

Food labels provide two very important information panels

regulated by the Food and Drug Administration: the ingredients list and the nutrition information panel. They're the same everywhere in the United States and very similar in Canada.

The ingredients list must contain all ingredients in descending order of content by weight. So, if a food lists salt or water or sugar first, you know that it is the highest-level ingredient in the product. Sometimes the manufacturer will disguise sugar by using several sources so that it can list something else as the first ingredient, and then corn syrup solids (corn sugar), glucose, and fructose follow. The ingredients list can tell you a great deal about a packaged food.

Although the major ingredients are at the top of the list, the bottom is just as important, because spices, enhancers like MSG, and other additives that can cause you trouble are used in small amounts. Learning to read the ingredients list is worth the time you invest, because you'll know what goes into the food you eat, and you can avoid questionable ingredients. Prevention is always the best medicine!

The nutrition information panel shows the serving size, calories, amount (in grams) of fat, carbohydrate, protein, amount (in milligrams) of cholesterol, sodium, potassium, and so on. It also contains information on vitamins and minerals as they contribute to the Recommended Daily Intake (RDI) for adults. Below the nutritional panel there is information on sodium, potassium, and carbohydrate, including fiber. Once you're familiar with the nutrition information panel, you'll be able to purchase one food in preference to another, using nutritional value as your guide.

I will take you through one food product, Post Bran Flakes, to illustrate these points. The ingredients list is about two-thirds of the way down on the right-side panel of the box when you're facing it.

> *Ingredients:* Whole grain wheat, wheat bran, sugar, corn syrup, salt, wheat flour, molasses, malted barley flour. BHT added to packaging material to preserve product freshness.

This ingredients list tells us that the product is good, but not as simple as you might think. The cereal is made mostly from wheat, wheat bran, and flour. The flavor is probably derived from molasses. The BHT in packaging is of no concern.

The nutritional label describes most of what we need to know. It tells us that a serving size is ¾ cup (30 grams), which delivers the following:

## Nutrition Facts

Serving Size ¾ cup (30g)
Servings Per Container about 15

| Amount Per Serving | Cereal | Cereal with ½ cup Skim Milk |
|---|---|---|
| **Calories** | 100 | 140 |
| Calories from Fat | 5 | 5 |
| | % Daily Value** | |
| **Total Fat** 0.5g* | 1% | 1% |
| Saturated Fat 0g | 0% | 0% |
| Polyunsaturated Fat 0g | | |
| Monounsaturated Fat 0g | | |
| **Cholesterol** 0mg | 0% | 0% |
| **Sodium** 220mg | 9% | 12% |
| **Potassium** 190mg | 5% | 11% |
| **Total Carbohydrate** 24g | 8% | 10% |
| Dietary Fiber 5g | 20% | 20% |
| Soluble fiber <1g | | |
| Insoluble fiber 4g | | |
| Sugars 6g | | |
| Other Carbohydrate 13g | | |
| **Protein** 3g | | |

*Amount in Cereal. One half cup skim milk contributes an additional 40 calories, 65mg sodium, 200mg potassium, 6g total carbohydrate (6g sugars), and 4g protein.
**Percent Daily values are based on a 2,000 calorie diet. Your daily values may be higher or lower depending on your calorie needs.

From this panel you can make a calculation. First, notice that the cereal delivers 5 calories from fat; that means it contains about ½ gram per serving, which is insignificant. The skim milk adds no fat. That means of the total 140 calories, fewer than 5 percent of calories come from fat.

The K-factor (potassium:sodium ratio) of the cereal is not good; that is, it contains more sodium than potassium. But with skim milk, it's a little better, so the product is okay for our purposes.

At the bottom of this panel is carbohydrate information. It's where we see how much complex carbohydrate and fiber are provided. You need at least 25 grams of fiber daily, and 30 grams is better. This cereal provides 5 grams of fiber per serving, which is meaningful, since 20 percent of any nutrient is significant but not overwhelming as in a cereal such as All Bran (which has 13 grams of fiber and would be more than 50 percent). Post Bran Flakes is a good source of fiber, and its fiber matrix has been broken down during processing, so it should be safe for most people.

To figure out how many calories in this cereal when used with skim milk are derived from carbohydrate, you need to know that ½ cup skim milk provides 4 grams of protein (not provided on the cereal label but on the milk panel). Since protein provides 4 calories per gram, this means that 16 calories of the 40 in skim milk (there is no fat in skim milk) are derived from protein, so the remaining 24 must come from milk sugar, lactose. Hence, the total carbohydrates are 24 grams or 96 calories (cereal) plus 6 grams (milk) or 24 calories for a total of 120 calories from carbohydrate (includes all sugars), which, when divided by 140, means that 86 percent of calories in a bowl of Post Bran Flakes made with skim milk are derived from carbohydrate. Lactose-intolerant people can usually tolerate about 7 grams of lactose; however, if you use soy beverage (soy milk) you avoid the issue altogether.

The ingredients list also names the vitamins and minerals that have been added. (I have not listed them here because

they are not important for this discussion.) There are no artificial colors or flavors in this particular cereal.

## Chemical Additives

While it's not so with Post Bran Flakes, at the bottom of
many ingredients lists are some chemical-sounding names:
erythroborate, EDTA, butylated hydroxytoluene (BHT),
propionic acid, monosodium glutamate (MSG), red dye no.
40, yellow dye no. 5, and others. These chemicals are used in
very small quantities; however, if you're sensitive to any one
of them, the amount doesn't matter. I cannot say they're un-
safe because their use is permitted by the FDA, but I avoid
them and I think you should as well.

The bran flakes in our example had BHT in the packaging material (usually in the box) to protect freshness. This is
not a concern since the box never actually comes in contact
with the cereal, which is protected by a liner.

## "Don't" Foods

Everyone I interviewed with IBD learns by trial and error
to avoid the following foods that cause flare-ups; some of
them have turned up in clinical research. Let me share them
with you. They'll appear again in other lists, but a little rep-
etition will make them that much more obvious to you.

The reason I say "some" have turned up in clinical studies
is because very few foods are actually studied clinically for
this purpose. To study foods for their flare-up potential
would be unreasonably costly and far too time consuming,
because the variations are too great. Therefore, when the
few that are tested confirm what we learn by experience, it
makes us realize that experience counts.

| | | |
|---|---|---|
| Chocolate of any type | Cabbage, uncooked | Blackberries |
| Beets | Fresh corn | Raspberries |
| Beet juice | Cooked corn | Grapes |

## "Do" Cereals

You should strive to get about 30 grams of fiber daily, of which at least 50 percent should be soluble fiber. Consequently, your choice of cereals is important. In Chapter Sixteen I list the level of fiber in a variety of cereals and other foods. Look them over to see what's available.

## Choosing a Breakfast Cereal

If a cereal doesn't provide more than 3 grams of fiber per serving, it's not acceptable. Be cautious with cereals that provide more than 6 grams of fiber per serving because they might contain unprocessed wheat bran. Reread the sections on the fiber matrix in Chapter Five. It's the fiber matrix, not the actual fiber, that's irritating. That's why the more processed bran cereals, such as bran flakes, oat flakes, and flax cereal, seem to be acceptable. Stick with cereals that are moderate in processed fiber, with from 3 to 6 grams per serving. If you want to experiment, do so with caution.

I've listed Corn Bran and corn cereals as "caution" cereals. Practically everyone I interviewed has difficulty with corn. However, their difficulty is most likely with the kernels of corn on the cob, not processed corn bran. Corn kernels have the intact matrix of the kernel; it's been removed in corn bran cereals. Corn Bran is a very good source of soluble fiber and it's worth trying, because if you can eat Corn Bran, you've got a moderate fiber source and a nourishing breakfast that tastes good, too.

## TABLE 6.1

### "Do" Cereals

---

#### *Cooked Cereals (Cook Thoroughly)*

| | |
|---|---|
| Barley | Oatmeal |
| Buckwheat | Ralston |
| Cream of Wheat | Wheatena |

#### *Cold (Ready-to-Eat) Cereals (Eat Mushy!)*

| | |
|---|---|
| Bran Flakes | Most |
| Shredded Wheat | Nutri-Grain |
| Flax cereal | Wheaties |

### "Caution" Cereals

---

| | |
|---|---|
| All-Bran | Corn cereals |
| Oat Bran | Fiber One |
| Corn Bran | |

## "Do" Vegetables

You should eat at least two vegetables with each meal, with the exception of breakfast (when you'll have fruit and fruit juice). I also suggest you eat one green salad or a cooked green vegetable such as spinach daily. If the salad ingredients are irritating, or you don't want to chance trying them, eat an additional serving of vegetables. Be cautious and experiment with salad ingredients to be sure they don't cause a flare-up; be especially careful of tomatoes, peppers, cucumbers, and other ingredients with skin or seeds because of the fiber matrix. One system that works is to use canned tomatoes on salads. Once you get past the idea, it's fine.

Vegetables provide excellent soluble dietary fiber and are the best sources of potassium, B vitamins, vitamin C, carotenoids, and minerals. Vegetable fiber is mostly soluble fiber, which helps prevent diarrhea, binds excess bile acids, and is seldom, if ever, irritating. Because of the fiber matrix, vegetable preparation is very important.

## Preparing Vegetables

It's important to peel any vegetables that have a defined skin, such as carrots, cucumbers, and potatoes. When eating baked vegetables, such as potatoes, squash, zucchini, and peppers, be sure to remove the skin after baking.

Cooking vegetables thoroughly in water or steam is as important as peeling them. The cooking method of choice is boiling in a moderate amount of fluid, and cooking should go far past crisp, all the way to soft. I realize this is contrary to what many dietitians and nutritionists recommend, but their advice is for people who don't have IBD.

Beans deserve special comment, because they contain excellent soluble fiber and one type of fiber—saponins—that is found almost nowhere else in similar abundance. They're nourishing in protein, vitamins, and minerals. A 1-cup serving of kidney beans, with its 225 calories, provides more than 15 grams of protein; that's over 20 percent of the RDI. About 72 percent of the calories in beans come from complex carbohydrate, and they provide more than 6 grams of soluble dietary fiber.

If cooked thoroughly, beans are okay for people with IBD. The best way I can describe their consistency when cooked correctly is "mushy." You can easily mash them and, when cool, spread them on bread if you desire. Bean cooking is easily accomplished without using excessive amounts of water. And when properly cooked, the beans will have a pasty consistency almost like peanut butter. A word of caution: Never use canned refried beans! Serve beans over steamed rice and you've got an excellent meal that provides 25 percent of your daily protein and fiber needs.

## Caution #1: Bean Salads

Bean salads are also appealing, but they're not for everyone. In my opinion, the tough fiber matrix of uncooked beans cannot be sufficiently broken down by the digestive system of many people. That's the first serious caution. The second caution is to be very careful with the oil selection. I suggest a high omega-3 oil, such as Puritan, walnut, or avocado, with a table-spoon of flax oil added. Olive oil is excellent, especially when flax oil is added, and is probably the best choice. However, using too much oil can cause a flare-up in some people. Remember the old saying "Better safe than sorry."

## Caution #2: Salad Bars

Salad bars are almost everywhere, in restaurants, super-markets, and delicatessens. There's only one problem: the fresh-looking lettuce, cherry tomatoes, broccoli, and other seemingly excellent produce may have been treated with sul-fate or preserved in another way to keep it looking fresh. It's hard to tell, and you seldom get a correct answer when you ask. It's not that waiters lie; they often don't know.

Even though sulfated foods look fresh and taste good, they can cause problems for people with inflammatory diseases like IBD. Only a good food diary will tell you what caused the trouble. That's why I urge you to keep a food diary that includes *where* you eat. It's often the only way you learn how you react to sulfated food.

A second caution for salad bars is all the potential for bowel irritation from peels and uncooked vegetables.

In Table 6.2 I've listed the best "Do" vegetables, "Caution" veg-etables, and a couple of "Don'ts." The "Don't" list is short, but the experiences of many people prove that it's very important.

### TABLE 6.2

#### "Do" Vegetables

| | |
|---|---|
| Asparagus | Broccoli |
| Avocado (also a fruit) | Butter beans |
| Beans (if canned, only with molasses or brown sugar, or thoroughly cooked) | Carrots |
| | Chard |
| Beans, white | Cowpeas |
| Black-eyed peas | Eggplant |

## "Do" Vegetables *(cont.)*

| | |
|---|---|
| Endive | Potatoes |
| Garbanzo beans (chickpeas) | Spinach |
| Green beans (Italian and snap) | Sweet potatoes |
| Kidney beans | Turnips |
| Lentils | Watercress |
| Lettuce | Wax beans |
| Lima beans | Winged beans |
| Mushrooms | Yam beans |
| Parsley | Yams |
| Peas | |

## "Caution" Vegetables

| | |
|---|---|
| Alfalfa sprouts | Kohlrabi |
| Artichokes | Mung bean sprouts |
| Bamboo shoots | Mustard greens |
| Brussels sprouts | Mustard spinach |
| Cabbage | Okra |
| Celery | Onions |
| Chickory | Peppers, bell |
| Chives | Pimientos |
| Collard greens | Pumpkin |
| Cucumber | Purslane |
| Fennel | Scallions |
| Garlic | Shallots |
| Gingerroot | Snow peas |
| Hominy | Squash |
| Jerusalem artichoke | Tomatoes |
| Kale | Yautia |

## "Don't" Vegetables

| | |
|---|---|
| Beets | Corn |

## "Do" Fruits

You can't eat too much fruit. Fruit has three advantages and one disadvantage. Except for avocados (they're actually pears), fruits contain no fat. Fruits provide quick energy in the form of the fruit sugars fructose and glucose. The soluble fiber in fruits modulates the way your body uses the fruit sugars, by slowing the rate at which they are absorbed. This slow absorption doesn't cause a rapid and large insulin response. The only disadvantage is that most fruits require peeling and, in citrus fruits such as oranges, the removal of the indigestible fibrous material around the pulp sections.

Juice made from whole fruits is excellent. It contains most of the soluble fiber, none of the skin or seeds, and is naturally sweet. Frozen concentrated juice is also good because the freeze-thaw cycle further breaks down any fiber matrix. In general, fruit juices are excellent potassium sources. The fiber in fruit juice makes the fruit's sugar acceptable, which is why high-pulp fruit juice is excellent for people with IBD. Read fruit juice labels to get a feeling for how they're made.

## Peel Fruits

If a fruit has a peelable skin, people with IBD should remove it before eating; otherwise, don't eat it! This need is obvious for apples, pears, peaches, kiwi, and citrus fruits, but who peels grapes or cherries? You may not be doing it, but you should! When it comes to peeling grape skins, you have to decide whether to develop the skill of a plastic surgeon and peel them with a sharp knife, learn to squeeze the inside of the grape into your mouth and throw the skin away, or avoid grapes entirely. Only you can decide which alternative is best.

## Section Citrus Fruits

Eating grapefruit, oranges, and other citrus fruits without triggering a flare-up seems to require careful removal of the white nondigestible, fibrous material around the sections and between the pulp and skin. This fibrous material (membrane or pith) can be irritating to sensitive intestinal tissues. It is quite noticeable in grapefruit, where it separates the edible sections. Be careful! The best thing to do is to remove it before eating. The fruit tastes much sweeter without it. The best chefs never leave the fibrous material on when serving a fruit dish with oranges. In addition to having a tough fiber matrix, which is troublesome, this material is rich in chemicals called bioflavonoids, some of which have been shown to have therapeutic value as antioxidants but others have been identified as irritants. My attitude is simple: Why take chances?

## Canned Fruits

Canned or jarred fruits are fine. Canned fruits have the skin removed (even from grapes), they've been cooked under pressure, and the hard fiber matrixes have often been broken down. Even the fibrous matrix has been removed from citrus fruits such as mandarin oranges and some grapefruit. The only drawback with canned fruits is the extra sugar in the syrup. You can pour or strain the syrup off and eat the fruit without it. Canned fruits are also available with no sugar added, canned in their own natural juices. This would be the better choice.

## "Don't" Fruits

You should avoid all dried fruits. Fruits (especially apricots) are dried with the skin intact, and bananas are dried when somewhat green. In addition, drying seems to toughen the fiber matrix and creates another problem from the protein-carbohydrate interaction called caramelization that didn't exist before.

Dried fruits are often sulfated to kill microorganisms and to preserve. Sulfated foods are notorious for causing flare-ups in people with inflammatory illnesses such as asthma, arthritis, psoriasis, and even allergies.

Cherries and grapes are usually eaten whole and not peeled. You should not eat them unless you're willing to peel them. Some berries (blackberries, boysenberries, and raspberries) can cause irritation because of their small seeds, so they should be avoided.

May "Don't" fruits are tolerated by some people, so I've also listed them as "Caution" fruits, but if you even suspect they don't agree with you, definitely eliminate them.

Table 6.3 identifies fruits that always seem safe—"Do" fruits. Certain fruits wear the "Caution" label, which means some people with IBD seem to have trouble with them because of the way they're prepared. "Don't" fruits include dried fruits, which are often sulfated, grapes, cherries, and berries that may cause irritation in some people.

## TABLE 6.3

### Fruits and Whole Juices

**"Do" Fruits**
**(Always Peel First)**

| | |
|---|---|
| Apples | Mangoes |
| Applesauce | Nectarines |
| Apricots | Oranges |
| Bananas | Papayas |
| Cantaloupes | Peaches |
| Casaba melons | Pears |
| Cranberries (jellied) | Persimmons |
| Honeydew melons | Plums |
| Lychees | |

**"Caution" Fruits**

| | |
|---|---|
| Blueberries | Lemons (peel) |
| Cherries (peel)* | Loganberries* |
| Cranberries* | Loquats |
| Currants | Mulberries* |
| Elderberries* | Pineapple |
| Gooseberries* | Strawberries* |
| Grapefruit (section) | Tangerines (peel and |
| Grapes (peel)* | section) |
| Jackfruit | Watermelon |
| Kiwifruit | |

*Eliminate these fruits if you suspect they don't agree with you.

### "Don't" Fruits

| | |
|---|---|
| Blackberries | Dried Fruits |
| Boysenberries | Grapes |
| Cherries | Raspberries |

## Eat Lots of Fish

Fish is one food that everyone rates high. IBD patients can usually eat fish without any flare-ups. So it seems you've got everything to gain and nothing to lose by making fish a staple in your diet.

In Chapter Fourteen I explain how the omega-3 oils in fish reduce inflammation and flare-ups, thus suppressing intestinal damage. With this in mind, I urge you to enjoy fish and explore the myriad ways in which it can be prepared (with the exception of frying).

## Omega-3 Oils

Table 6.4 lists finfish as "high," "moderate," and "low" in omega-3 oil content. High means from 1.5 to 3 grams of omega-3 oils per standard 3½-ounce serving; medium means from 1 to 2 grams of omega-3 oils per serving; and low means less than 1.5 grams per serving. I urge you to keep omega-3 oil content in mind when you eat fish. Much excellent research proves these oils prevent inflammation. They also reduce the risk of breast and ovarian cancers.

## TABLE 6.4

### Finfish: High Omega-3 Oils

| | |
|---|---|
| Anchovy | Mullet |
| Dogfish | Sablefish |
| Eel | Salmon |
| Herring | Trout |
| Mackerel | |

### Finfish: Moderate Omega-3 Oils

| | |
|---|---|
| Bluefish | Smelt |
| Carp | Sturgeon |
| Catfish | Tuna |
| Sea trout | Whitefish |

### Finfish: Low Omega-3 Oils

| | |
|---|---|
| Bass | Perch |
| Cod | Pike |
| Dolphinfish | Plaice |
| Drum | Pompano |
| Flounder | Shark |
| Grouper | Sheepshead |
| Hake | Sole |
| Halibut | Swordfish |

In addition to the oil content, the texture of fish provides another advantage. Red meat is not acceptable for people with IBD because of irritation from undigestible fibrous parts. We call this material gristle, which is part of the tendon's tough blood vessels and membranes. It seems characteristic of all meat, including game. No counterpart exists in fish. Indeed, cooked fish can usually be cut with a fork or even pulled apart with a spoon, which illustrates my point. Of course, beware of bones!

## Cooking Fish

Fish can be baked, boiled, broiled, poached, dried, and even eaten raw. Just don't fry it, or bread it and fry it. "I can't eat fried fish" was the universal comment of IBD people I interviewed. I believe the trouble comes from materials created in the frying process, when local high temperatures are created that can alter the structure of many substances. When protein (fish) and carbohydrate (bread) are cooked together, a reaction between the two can produce tough, undigestible material. That explains why breaded and fried fish should be avoided, and also suggests that dried fish could pose a problem.

## Fish Economics

Pound for pound, fish is more expensive than red meat. But a pound-for-pound comparison is deceptive, because it doesn't account for the protein and calories in each. If you think in terms of purchasing protein per calorie, most fish usually provides more than twice as much protein as meat. For example, 3 ounces of halibut provides 22 grams of protein in 119 calories; 3 ounces of lean ground beef provides 22 grams of protein in 219 calories. That means that if you're seeking nutrition from your food dollar, fish provides about twice as much, even though it might cost more. Meat yields twice the calories for the same amount of protein, and the calories from meat are the worst kind—saturated fat, which favors inflammation!

## Frozen Fish

Modern fishing fleets have shipboard facilities to fillet, cut into steaks, and flash-freeze fish. Consequently, frozen fish usually has a nutritional edge, and the omega-3 oils are preserved in the process. Frozen fresh whole fish, fillets, and steaks are excellent.

## Canned Fish

Select fish packed in brine or water if possible; otherwise, drain off the oil. Canned tuna and salmon are excellent sources of protein and the omega-3 oils, and actually cost less than fresh. Use mayonnaise sparingly because it's high in the wrong kind of fat and has a poor K-factor. Alternatively, low-fat mayonnaise is fine (except for its poor K-factor).

# Mollusks, Crustaceans, and Cephalopods

I have never encountered any "Don't" finfish for people with IBD. However, mollusks (oysters, clams, etc.), crustaceans (shrimp, crabs, etc.), and cephalopods (squid, octopus, etc.) fall into the "Don't" category. The one exception seems to be scallops. Many respondents expressed difficulty with one or all of the foods in this grouping, and clinical research supports their observations. If you can eat them, they are good protein sources and are loaded with vitamins and minerals. However, they don't supply many omega-3 oils, so they don't have the inflammation-fighting dietary impact of finfish.

In addition, mollusks, crustaceans, and cephalopods have many tough fibrous or shell-like materials that irritate sensitive bowels. Therefore, people who said this type of seafood caused a flare-up could simply be describing the result of irritation, not some type of allergy or sensitivity. Because most people with IBD can eat scallops (not fried, of course), I would expect scallops to appear on the list of troublesome products if an allergy or sensitivity was involved, but they don't. As you can see in Table 6.5, most other forms of seafood have very low levels of omega-3 oils.

## TABLE 6.5

### "Don't" or "Great Caution" Seafood

*Other Seafood: Low Omega-3 Oils*

| | |
|---|---|
| Abalone | Mussel |
| Clam | Octopus |
| Conch | Oysters |
| Crab | Shrimp |
| Lobster | Squid |

## Eat Poultry and Fowl Weekly

Chicken, turkey, pheasant, guinea fowl, squab, and other birds are low in fat and excellent sources of protein. Select only the breast and other light meat (which is especially good and nonirritating) and avoid the dark meat and wings. Because dark meat comes from active muscles (specifically legs), it's abundant with gristle that remains undigested, so it should be avoided.

Breast from waterfowl is mostly dark meat, which is free of irritating factors, but it should be eaten with caution. The breast of ducks or geese is definitely acceptable.

## Cooking Poultry

Bake, broil, barbecue, or boil poultry for use in salads; avoid breading and frying, or even just frying. Try to remove the skin before cooking; however, the skin is frequently left on during cooking, especially when roasting, to impart more moisture and flavor to the meat. In that case, ALWAYS *remove the skin after cooking*. The skin causes intestinal irritation and provides the wrong kind of fat.

The major problem with making chicken or turkey salad is the mayonnaise. It doesn't agree with some people's digestive tracts and contains the wrong oils. There are two solutions to this problem. Plain yogurt or a ripe avocado is an excellent medium for diced or shredded poultry. Although an avocado has a fat content similar to that of mayonnaise, it's a rich source of unsaturated oils and contains some omega-3 oils. Yogurt is similarly low in fat and provides calcium. Sometimes a creamy, mildly seasoned salad dressing made from polyunsaturated oil is excellent. You can always add a tablespoon of flax oil.

## *Don't* Take Out Fast-food Chicken

Don't eat fast-food fried chicken. Fast-food chicken is a high-fat, high-sodium, excessively spiced food trap. It's definitely a "Don't" food.

## Avoid Processed Poultry

Turkey versions of salami, bologna, frankfurters, and other traditional beef products are available in most supermarkets. Advertising creates the illusion that they're better for you by suggesting they are low-fat versions of their beef counterparts. This is truly an illusion, because they're almost as high in the wrong kind of fat as the beef version, and they usually contain artificial flavors, colors, excessive salt, and preservatives as well. Calculate the calories from protein, fat, and carbohydrate from one of these products, and then compare your results with regular turkey or chicken and all-beef or pork versions of the same product—you're in for a surprise.

The ideal turkey or chicken breast purchased in the supermarket is wrapped in its own skin. Simply remove it before or after slicing.

## Red Meat: Once Monthly—Why Not Stop Altogether?

Since I first wrote *Eating Right for a Bad Gut,* much research has been done on inflammation in general, and in IBD specifically. There is no doubt that by shifting your dietary fat balance (Chapters Thirteen and Fourteen) you can reduce inflammation. However, it calls for reducing to a minimum all animal fat, especially from red meat. The best approach is simply to stop eating red meat, or eat it only once a month.

Other epidemiological research indicates that eating beef in particular, and high-cholesterol meat in general, predisposes a person to IBD. This finding is consistent with beef's ability to make people susceptible to other inflammatory diseases and several types of cancer. Obviously, eating it once a month is safe and prudent, although there are several excellent reasons to cut out red meat altogether. Red meat seems to always make the list of foods that cause flare-ups. The saturated fat of red meat is the basis of heart disease and the inflammatory prostaglandins. From an environmental standpoint, raising beef depletes many resources.

If those reasons aren't enough, red meat also seems to irritate the intestinal tract in people with IBD. I believe this irritation comes from the gristle, because ground meat is easier to tolerate. However, ground meat is often a poor choice because it is always higher in fat than other cuts.

Occasionally I'll meet a person with IBD who can eat red meat, so I don't want to be overly pessimistic. My admonition is to eat red meat once a month, as in Mediterranean diets. People who eat this way generally have less heart disease and cancer, and more recent studies show they have less IBD, multiple sclerosis, and rheumatoid arthritis.

## *Don't* Eat Organ Meats

Organ meats are high in the worst kinds of fat. If there's any single group of foods that clearly belongs in the "Don't" category, it's beef, lamb, and pork organ meats.

## *Don't* Eat Processed Meats

Avoid all processed meats, such as bologna, salami, frank-furters, and sausages. They're excessive in saturated fat and full of nitrates, preservatives, spices, and salt. Most people avoid processed meats because they cause flare-ups; they favor inflammation and are not good for your heart and arteries.

## Cooking Meat

Broiling and roasting meat are definitely safe methods. Barbecuing appears to be all right for some people if the meat isn't charred. Any kind of rare meat seems to present a problem, probably because some of the membrane material can't be digested until it's cooked. Therefore, meat should be cooked at least until it's pink; in a restaurant, a chef would call it "medium." Never fry meat, since any fried food causes a serious problem.

Portion size is important. Because many people are sensitive to something in meat, the amount eaten must exceed a threshold to trigger a reaction. Many people I interviewed said, "As long as I eat a small portion and chew it well, there's no problem." Therefore, the best rule is to play it safe and choose small servings.

## TABLE 6.6

### "Do" Meat (Eat Once Monthly)

| | |
|---|---|
| Beef (lean) | Rabbit |
| Ham (lean) | Veal |
| Lamb (fat trimmed) | Venison |
| Pork (fat removed) | |

### "Caution" Meats

| | |
|---|---|
| Filets | Lamb chops (fat trimmed) |
| Flank steak | Prime rib of beef |
| Ground chuck | |

### "Don't" Meats

| | |
|---|---|
| Organ meats | Sandwich spreads from meat |
| Processed meats | Sausages |

## Do Eat Pasta

Eating pasta is an excellent way to obtain both protein and complex carbohydrate. Read the ingredients list to be sure the first ingredient is wheat or spinach. Corn pasta is probably all right, though not widely available.

## With Pasta, Sauce Is King

With pasta, sauce is king and that's where you should be careful. Most people can eat peeled, cooked tomatoes, but the spices used in a sauce can be a problem. Therefore, select mild spices and use onions, shallots, garlic, and ginger carefully and sparingly. Avoid using a condiment such as garlic directly; instead, use a little garlic oil made by crushing fresh garlic. Do the same with a small amount of onion or shallots (which should be finely chopped and boiled first) to get the flavor. Put the sauce through a food processor or ricer after cooking to blend it and make it smooth. Try freezing a sauce after it has been prepared. Freezing preserves the nutrition and breaks down the fiber matrix even more.

Tomato sauce is important for your health. The antioxidants help prevent the tissue damage that comes with a flare-up and possibly without one. Men and women who eat tomato sauce regularly have a lower risk of colon cancer, and men have a markedly reduced prostate cancer risk. So there are reasons besides controlling IBD for eating pasta with tomato sauce.

An excellent meal is pasta with a tomato sauce containing fish or poultry. Tomato sauces with broccoli, zucchini, carrots, or mushrooms are also excellent. Just be sure the vegetables are cooked correctly, and use the food processor after preparation. Parmesan cheese adds both flavor and some calcium. *Bon appétit!*

## Use Garlic, Onions, Chives, and Shallots with Caution

These foods are good for you, and you should be able to eat them. They help protect us from cancer, high blood pressure, high blood sugar, and other illnesses. However, a number of people claim they cause flare-ups. When you use these foods (for example, in a tomato sauce), cook them thoroughly in water and then use the water and the pureed bulb. This works because you've broken down the fiber matrix, while flavoring your sauce with the liquid.

## Be Cautious with Dairy Products

Dairy products are a mixed blessing: they're nourishing, but they can cause problems. Many people, like Jean, express the problem very clearly: "Milk causes serious intestinal discomfort, gas, bloating, and spasms. Lactaid makes it possible for me to use milk on cereal."

This typical response brings to the fore the most common problem with milk: many people with IBD are lactose intolerant.

Do try to use nonfat dairy products, such as cottage cheese and yogurt made from skim or nonfat milk, and keep a food diary to identify any problems.

## Dairy Desserts

Sherbet seems to be well tolerated by all people with IBD, and some can eat low-fat ice cream. But many people identified standard ice cream as a cause of flare-ups, so it should be eaten with great caution.

Pudding made with skim or Lactaid milk is an excellent dessert. Let's do some arithmetic: ½ cup butterscotch pudding made from a mix with low-fat milk contains 4.7 grams of fat; that's 42 calories from fat out of a total of 171 calories, or only 25 percent from fat. Add some fruit, such as ripe bananas, and you've reduced the fat to less than 20 percent of calories. You can improve it even more by using skim milk. It's a nourishing dessert. Finally, try making puddings with soy or rice beverage.

## Never Eat Nuts

Most people have difficulty digesting nuts. I suspect bits of nuts irritate the lining of the intestine. Other research on the digestibility of nuts indicates that these bits go through the system intact in all people, not just those with IBD. Nuts cause more food sensitivities and allergies than any other food category, which is one more reason for caution.

# CHAPTER 7

# Sensible Vitamin and Mineral Supplements

To function normally, your body requires nineteen vitamins and minerals daily in addition to protein, fat, carbohydrates, and fiber. These requirements are expressed in terms of the recommended daily intake (RDI) and are often very small (trace) quantities. For example, every day you need just 400 micrograms (400 millionths of a gram) of folic acid (a B vitamin), an amount contained in a tiny dot. A consistent shortage can cause serious health problems.

People with IBD face a special challenge getting enough folic acid. Drugs prescribed to quiet your intestine, such as Azulfidine, interfere with folic-acid absorption. As if that were not a sufficient challenge to your health, diarrhea increases the loss of folic acid along with other nutrients. A shortfall in folic acid not only compromises your health on a daily basis but also increases your risk of colon and other cancers.

Pregnant women are especially susceptible to folic-acid shortfall, because not only does their need increase dramatically, but more is required to support the growing fetus. Indeed, the most common birth defects (neural tube defects, such as cleft palate), which occur during the first eight weeks of pregnancy, are traced to a folic-acid shortfall, and about 93 percent are prevented by taking supplements. The prevention of both cancer and birth defects illustrates the need for sensible supplementation for most people, especially anyone with IBD.

In contrast, calcium is required in comparatively large amounts, ranging from 1,000 milligrams (or 1 gram) for men and most women up to menopause, when it increases to 1,500 milligrams—and some experts call for 2,000 milligrams. Magnesium's requirement is somewhere in the middle; you need 400 milligrams (four-tenths of a gram) daily. With the exception of calcium (which will be discussed in detail in Chapter Twenty-two) and magnesium, all your vitamin and mineral needs can be packed into one or two single large tablets. I don't believe in leaving anything to chance, so I recommend that you ensure your diet with supplementation to avoid any possible marginal deficiencies.

Having IBD makes eating a balanced diet very unlikely. I am always impressed by the way IBD patients learn to avoid foods that cause discomfort; however, forgoing meat, shellfish, and many vegetables means B vitamins, vitamin A, iron, zinc, and magnesium are likely to be in short supply. Discomfort caused by dairy products makes getting sufficient calcium and magnesium difficult, if not impossible. This doesn't mean that people with IBD will fall outside the RDI safety net; rather, it means they are more vulnerable to dietary imbalance and shortfall than average people. Add medication to the mix and the nutrient shortfalls become serious. Having IBD is an excellent case for sensible supplementation.

## Malabsorption

Ongoing watery stools, not to mention severe diarrhea, living with intestinal inflammation, or having had part of the small intestine and colon removed creates a serious likelihood of below-average absorption of many, if not all, nutrients from food. One proven way to overcome this possible shortfall is simply to add more nutrients. Technology makes this easy through vitamin and mineral supplements.

# Medication

Some IBD patients I interviewed take as many as twenty pills daily, covering ten or more different medications. Even the most common medication, aspirin, increases the need for vitamin C and folic acid, so people with IBD need to think seriously about the effects of the medications they take. Just consider the side effects people describe: dizziness, light-headedness, drowsiness, dry mouth, dry eyes, nausea, moon face, and lethargy, to name a few. If your doctor doesn't believe drug side effects are physiologically important, ask if he or she believes they account for more stress, which would increase nutrient need.

## Look to the Experts

Two surveys of registered dietitians showed that 50 to 60 percent of them supplemented their diets. About 45 percent of the average population use supplements. What do dietitians know that the rest of us don't? They probably realize they don't eat a balanced diet! After all, most of them are women and eat fewer than 2,000 calories daily; they simply don't want to leave health to chance.

Another, more recent, study of supplement use showed that the more educated people are, the more likely they are to use supplements. Use is also proportional to income.

## Common Questions About Supplement Use

*Aren't excess vitamins and minerals just excreted, making expensive urine?*

Even if you're starving, your body will lose some vitamins and minerals daily through excretion. Under those conditions, your urine is truly "expensive." If your blood levels of nutrients are high, the levels in your urine will also be higher; that's normal human physiology.

*What's the upper limit of safety for vitamins and minerals?*

Up to about ten times the RDI of vitamins (excepting A and D) and minerals (excepting zinc and selenium) is safe in normal people. Most are safe at many times that level.

*Isn't it expensive to take vitamins and minerals?*

Our society spends about $1.00 per capita daily on soft drinks. Is that wasteful? The average adult woman spends $1.00 daily on her hair. Is that wasteful? Expensive is only meaningful by comparison. The supplements in this program are less than 75 cents daily and only a few would reach $1.00. You've got to ask yourself: "Is my health worth it?"

## Nutrition Insurance

"Nutrition insurance" is an overworked slogan, but here it is appropriate. I would like you to supplement your diet with at least one-half (50 percent) of the RDI for all nineteen vitamins and minerals—I would prefer 100 percent in view of IBD's effect on health. Why this amount? The diet plan proposed in Part II will supply the RDI for most of the required nutrients; however, our major dietary objective is to reduce inflammation and stop flare-ups; as a result, some variety is lost and some nutrients will fall short. Supplementation is an easy way of ensuring that the nutrients are present in adequate supply and any excess will be additional insurance.

Use a supplement that provides the vitamins and minerals and amounts listed in Table 7.1. Most supplements will contain within 10 to 20 percent of the values listed here. It is important for your supplement to contain all these vitamins and minerals. It is essential that you get them daily.

# TABLE 7.1

## Basic Supplement

| Nutrient | Amount per Tablet* | Percent U.S. RDI |
|---|---|---|
| | ***Vitamins*** | |
| Vitamin A (as beta-carotene) | 2,500 IU** (500 mcg RE***) | 50 |
| Vitamin D | 200 IU (5 mcg) | 50 |
| Vitamin E | 15 IU (5 mg alphatocopherol equivalents) | 50 |
| Vitamin C | 30 mg | 50 |
| Folic acid | 0.2 mg | 50 |
| Thiamin (B₁) | 0.75 mg | 50 |
| Riboflavin (B₂) | 0.86 mg | 50 |
| Niacin | 10 mg | 50 |
| Vitamin B₆ | 1 mg | 50 |
| Vitamin B₁₂ | 3 mcg | 50 |
| Biotin | 0.15 mg (150 mcg) | 50 |
| Pantothenic acid | 5 mg | 50 |
| | ***Minerals*** | |
| Calcium | 125 mg | 25 |
| Phosphorus | 180 mg | 40 |
| Iodine | 75 mcg | 50 |
| Iron | 9 mg | 50 |
| Magnesium | 50 mg | 12.5 |
| Copper | 1 mg | 50 |
| Zinc | 1 mg | 50 |
| Selenium | 50 mcg | **** |
| Manganese | 0.5 mg | **** |
| Chromium | 50 mcg | **** |
| Molybdenum | 30 mcg | **** |

*Two tablets provide 100 percent U.S. RDI for all nutrients except calcium, phosphorus, and magnesium; see text for explanation.
**International Units.
***Microgram retinol equivalents.
****U.S. RDI not established.

Few products satisfy the preceding criteria exactly, but those that don't are probably fine. Usually the product you select will have less calcium and magnesium. Do not worry about that because you should take extra amounts of these two minerals anyway, as I will discuss later. Your diet already contains excess phosphorus and about 20 percent of the magnesium you need. If the product you select comes to within 20 percent of the calcium, magnesium, and phosphorus listed in Table 7.1, it is fine. Don't select a supplement that varies in these areas by more than that amount. Products that meet my criteria are labeled to deliver 100 percent of the U.S. RDI in a two-tablet serving.

## Is More Better?

Anyone with IBD should take two tablets of the supplement in Table 7.1; in fact, I believe three would be appropriate in most cases. I estimate that I personally get about 70 to 100 percent of the RDI of most vitamins, but not all minerals, from my food. So I take two tablets daily, or 100 percent of the U.S. RDI. The excess, probably up to 200 percent of the U.S. RDI or even more, is completely safe; the extra will do no harm, and there's much evidence that says the excess will do much good.

Except for vitamins A and D, vitamins are safe at ten or more times the RDI, so if you choose to do as I do and take some extra, you don't have to worry, as you're not harming yourself. Recent studies of elderly people indicate that as we age our needs increase, so if you're over 40, taking more than the RDI is undoubtedly good. The reason we are discovering these needs now is that people are living longer, and early nutrition research was usually conducted on college-age volunteers.

There's much evidence to suggest that IBD patients need more vitamin E, everyone needs up to 500 milligrams of vitamin C daily, and calcium is definitely a special case. Part II will make these needs more apparent.

## Calcium

Adult women require 1,000 milligrams of calcium each day up to about menopause, when most experts believe that calcium intake should be elevated to 1,500 milligrams—some say 2,000. Milk, yogurt, and cheese are the most common sources of calcium; however, a 1-cup serving of broccoli or spinach provides the calcium of a half glass of milk, together with other nutrients. So you should ask yourself if you consume sufficient dairy products and calcium-rich foods each day. Common sense, and now even the government, says to use about 1,000 to 1,200 milligrams of calcium supplements daily.

### Food Sources for 1,000 Milligrams of Calcium

| Food | Amount | Calories | Comments |
|------|--------|----------|----------|
| Cheddar cheese | 5.0 oz | 560 | Fat is bad |
| Low-fat cottage cheese | 5.2 oz | 1,066 | Too much fat and sodium |
| Skim milk | 27 fl oz (3⅓ 8-oz glasses) | 290 | Good source |
| Low-fat yogurt | 19 oz | 466 | Good source |
| Fortified orange juice | 27 fl oz (3⅓ 8-oz glasses) | 400 | Excellent source High potassium |

Most government nutrition and food analyses indicate that calcium is generally short in most of our diets. Nearly all experts on the subject both use and recommend calcium supplements. In addition to the difficulty of obtaining adequate dietary calcium, many lifestyle habits, such as caffeine use, excess sodium intake, and lack of exercise, also cause calcium loss.

Calcium shortfalls, unlike those of most nutrients, are additive. If you fall short for a year or two when you're a teenager, and then fall short again during your adult and childbearing years (for women), you will have less dense bones than if you hadn't fallen short at all. Below-normal bone density is a disease called osteoporosis, which causes much suffering and even death in old age.

Bone calcium loss is accelerated by caffeine (coffee, tea, soft drinks), excess red meat, salt, and inadequate exercise. However, much worldwide clinical research has proven that bone density can be restored by using calcium supplements. If you drink more than 2 cups of coffee or its equivalent as tea or soft drinks (10 cups or cans daily), take an extra 200 milligrams daily. Exercise is essential for everyone.

## Magnesium: A Partner with Calcium

Most dietary analyses indicate that we usually also fall short in the mineral magnesium. Since 200 to 400 milligrams of magnesium are required daily, it, like calcium, doesn't fit into a single tablet. Therefore, a good policy is to take a calcium supplement that also contains some magnesium.

Some self-proclaimed experts advise a specific calcium-magnesium ratio for good health. However, a brilliant scientist, Dr. Mildred Seelig, conducted a careful study of adult needs for calcium and magnesium and proved that once you take in about 400 milligrams of magnesium daily, the body can use all the calcium it gets very effectively, and there is no need to get more magnesium.

## Iron

Iron is another special case. A typical diet contains about 6 milligrams of iron for each 1,000 calories. Women require 15 milligrams each day. This translates to almost 3,000 calories. Few women consume more than 2,000 calories each day, hence the shortfall, and it's worse if you've got IBD. Even after menopause, when a woman's iron requirement drops to that of men (10 milligrams a day), most don't get enough in food. To add insult to injury, research has proved that some IBD patients do not absorb iron effectively; therefore, making sure you get enough is simply common sense. The multiple vitamin-mineral supplement I propose will handle this nicely. If you need more iron, a simple blood test will reveal it.

## B-Complex Vitamins

Some people feel better if they use the B-complex vitamins as a supplement over and above the basic supplement I recommend. The B vitamins are those listed in Table 7.1 as folic acid, thiamin (B$_1$), riboflavin (B$_2$), niacin, vitamin B$_6$ (sometimes listed as pyridoxal phosphate), vitamin B$_{12}$, biotin, and pantothenic acid. If you wish to take more B vitamins, always take them together as a supplement containing all the B vitamins balanced in the same RDI levels, and never take more than 400 percent (or four times) of the RDI in a single tablet.

## Special Supplements of Single Nutrients

There is a continuing debate surrounding vitamins C and E, beta-carotene, zinc, and a few other nutrients.

*Vitamin C:* This is one of the most abused vitamins. The government recommends 65 milligrams each day, and other expert nutritionists recommend up to a gram. The medications most commonly used in the treatment of IBD sometimes destroy vitamin C; therefore, getting enough is an important consideration.

There's a debate among those who advocate taking up to 10 grams per day and those who advise caution and using no more than the U.S. RDI of 65 milligrams. This debate has precipitated much discussion among experts and will probably continue into the next century. The lack of resolution has to do with the criteria on which RDIs are established. Not long ago scurvy was the deficiency disease of vitamin C, but now we are considering such weighty issues as its role in preventing cancer and heart disease.

In the past, it was suggested that vitamin C had some specific relationship to IBD. In Part II you will learn about inflammation and the substances that cause it, as well as the tissue damage that is one of the results. Tissue damage can be suppressed with antioxidants, and vitamin C is one of nature's best antioxidants; in fact, our body depends on it. For this reason, an extra 500 to 1,000 milligrams of vitamin C is appropriate. In addition, some drugs used to suppress inflammation cause vitamin C loss.

The IBD diet recommended in Part II provides at least 100 milligrams of vitamin C, depending on your use of fruits, vegetables, and grains. In the opinion of many experts, an additional vitamin C supplement of up to 1,000 milligrams daily does no harm and can do much good.

**Vitamin E:** Vitamin E does seem to have an effect on IBD beyond its importance in maintaining general good health. During inflammation, free radical reactions initiated by leukotrienes (see Chapter Ten) cause damage that vitamin E can suppress. A free radical is an unstable compound with an extra electron or proton that reacts readily with other molecules. In IBD, free radical reactions accompany inflammation and cause tissue damage. In other tissues these reactions cause damage that can lead to cancer. Free radical reactions are stopped by antioxidants, of which vitamin E is the most ubiquitous and most effective.

Careful clinical studies at the Medical College in London, England, established that vitamin E helps prevent tissue damage during inflammation. Unfortunately, researchers found that in tissues where it is needed most, vitamin E levels fall far below normal. You don't need a medical degree to conclude that a daily vitamin E supplement makes sense.

In addition, the vitamin E requirement is also proportional to polyunsaturated fat intake; research has proven that vitamin E supplements reduce the risk of heart disease.

If you follow this diet plan and use the basic supplement, you should exceed the RDI for vitamin E. In my opinion, it makes sense to take more vitamin E: at least 100 IU daily, and 400 IU daily would be better. Recent research indicates that people at risk of heart disease can benefit from 800 IU of vitamin E daily (a level impossible to get from food).

**Selenium:** This trace mineral is generally short in people with IBD, because they don't eat sufficient selenium-containing fruits, vegetables, shellfish, and meat.

Folk wisdom teaches that we should eat an apple a day. Although the originator of that advice probably didn't have selenium in mind, it turns out that apples are an excellent selenium source. By eating a variety of fruits, vegetables, and grains, you obtain ample selenium—and, for insurance, use the basic vitamin-mineral supplement described in Table 7.1. If you take an additional vitamin E supplement, select one that also contains 25 to 50 micrograms of selenium.

**Zinc:** Dietary studies have indicated that many IBD sufferers have inadequate zinc partly because their diets lack variety (especially meat and shellfish) and partly from malabsorption. There is no indication that people with IBD should self-medicate with zinc tablets, but a multiple vitamin-mineral supplement that provides up to 100 percent of the U.S. RDI for zinc is safe and effective. Zinc taken in amounts five to ten times the RDI should be monitored by a physician, because it can cause a change in cholesterol metabolism. The recommended supplement in Table 7.1 will provide adequate zinc.

**Beta-carotene:** Beta-carotene is the vegetable precursor of vitamin A; consequently, our body converts beta-carotene to vitamin A as it is required for bodily function. Studies of dietary adequacy usually indicate that most people, especially those over 50, get less vitamin A or beta-carotene than they require. The diet in Part II should be adequate in beta-carotene, especially if you use the recommended supplement.

## Using EPA Supplements

Eicosapentaenoic acid (EPA), an essential omega-3 oil, is a polyunsaturated fatty acid that is found in fish, green plants, some seeds, and nuts that grow on trees. Clinical studies of EPA are reviewed in Part II, and I recommend a supplement of 2 to 3 grams daily. However, EPA supplements are relatively new, so they must be consumed with care. Divide 2,000 by the number of milligrams of EPA and alpha linolenic acid (ALA) in each capsule to get the number of capsules necessary to obtain 1 gram. For example, suppose your EPA capsules contain 180 milligrams of EPA and 100 milligrams of ALA; 2,000 divided by 280 yields 7.1, which we round to 7; so 7 is the number of capsules necessary to get 2 grams (2,000 milligrams) of EPA. Larger capsules often provide more than 180 milligrams of EPA; however, the larger capsule might be difficult to swallow.

Most EPA is sold as a concentrate from fish oil, which contains DHA as well. DHA (short for docosahexaenoic acid) is also an important nutrient, but it has no known effect on either IBD or other inflammatory problems. However, DHA does have an important role in the metabolism of EPA.

Don't be confused by the size of the capsule or the percentage concentration. Simply look for the EPA and ALA content in milligrams per capsule and take enough to get at least 1 gram each day. Up to 3 grams of EPA daily is safe and effective.

## Evening Primrose and Black Currant Oil: Gamma Linolenic Acid (GLA)

You will learn in Part II that a diet that contains omega-3 oils, such as EPA and flax oils, can prevent inflammation and make any flare-ups milder. Juxtaposed in this metabolic process is another oil called gamma linolenic acid (GLA). This oil helps to modulate inflammation, and you can take it as a supplement. I consider GLA optional, and if you decide to take it, you need to take only one capsule (1 gram) daily. It can be purchased as either Evening Primrose Oil or Black Currant Oil.

## Additional Supplements

The practice of food supplementation has grown slowly in the United States, from its beginnings in the late 1920s and 1930s. Today, it ranges from the modest multiple vitamin-mineral supplement, which I recommend as a foundation, to all types of single supplements and combinations of various nutrients.

People use specific supplements, such as vitamins C and E, because they make them feel better, or as preventives for heart disease and cancer. Give the diet in Part II and its recommended supplements a reasonable chance. Extensive clinical research has proven that it takes a good three months to get maximum results. Remember my saying: "Nutrition works in slow motion."

---

## Supplements Recap

The diet plan in Part II is nutritionally sound, with the exception of moderate shortfalls in iron, calcium, magnesium, and a few vitamins. However, people with IBD require more of these and other nutrients, and a multiple vitamin-mineral supplement is essential for nutrition insurance.

# CHAPTER 8

# *Medicinal Foods*

Research has confirmed (see references for this chapter at the end of the book) that it is preferable to bring a flare-up into remission without drugs (specifically steroids). It is better if you can bring it into remission at home without being hospitalized for either enteral nutrition (EN) or total parenteral nutrition (TPN). In addition to vitamins and minerals, some individuals, especially children, also need specialized foods to support a diet short in calories, protein, and electrolytes. Medicinal foods are the answer.

Although these foods can be used at any time to add nutrition, they are especially helpful under special circumstances, even if boring. Most of them can completely sustain life. I should point out that *medicinal foods* is a descriptive term I like to use; however, they're often described as supplemental foods. Don't confuse them with what health-food faddists call "nutraceuticals" and "nutrafoods."

## What Are Supplemental Foods?

Typically, medicinal-supplemental foods come in the form of prepared drinks, drink mixes, frozen shakes, and puddings. They are designed to deliver calories, protein, vitamins, minerals, and balanced electrolytes. Calories are usually provided as both fat and carbohydrate.

Some products use both vegetable and dairy protein sources, while many are completely lactose free. Fat in these foods is derived from excellent sources (often medium-chain triglycerides) that are easily absorbed and excellent for your health. Everyone needs calories, and digestible fat is fine.

The products—Nutra/Shakes, Great Shake, etc.—mentioned below and in Table 8.1 also provide a good, if not excellent, potassium-sodium balance along with all the nutrition. Some of them are "low residue," meaning that they are predigested and rely very little on the digestive system. Others provide varying levels of protein that must be digested, or even some dietary fiber.

## Suppose You Simply Need to Gain Weight

When you can't gain weight, or if you've got chronic, watery stools, or suffer from both conditions, like many of the people I meet, you're losing some nourishment, including calories, through those stools. You may be vulnerable to malnutrition because of malabsorption. You will always do best by eating many small meals, and medicinal-supplemental foods can be a very effective way to improve your health, give you more energy, and add pounds.

People who tolerate lactose can choose from a variety of convenient products that include Nutra/Shakes and Great Shake. These products are convenient frozen milk shakes that pack 230 calories, with excellent nutrition, into 4 ounces. They nearly meet the criteria for an ideal food supplement and provide calories, protein, and electrolytes.

Two snacks each day from any one of these products will provide about 500 calories, 40 percent of your daily protein, and 40 to 60 percent of your nutrient requirements; they are balanced with a good K-factor for sodium and potassium. They make getting balanced nutrition easy and enjoyable.

Recovery Power Foods are designed for people who are recovering from surgery or may not be eating correctly for many reasons. While not designed specifically for IBD, they are excellent if you can tolerate them. They come in easily made shakes as well as in bar form. They are especially good for children, and the nutrition delivery is excellent.

## Special Products for Children

Pedia Sure is made for children 1 to 10 years old, but it can be used at any age because it is an excellent balance of the essential oils as well as other nutrients. Children with IBD often fail to grow as they should simply because they aren't eating enough food, and Pedia Sure can be the answer. Supplying all the growth nutrients and calories, it comes in varied flavors with and without fiber.

Remember that pound for pound, children and adolescents need more calories than adults. Relax the normal instinct that drives us to feed children nutritious foods, and instead try to make the food they eat nutritious. Use the medicinal-supplement foods I've described in this chapter. A good trick that adds both calories and omega-3 oils is to add a little flax oil to the shake and blend it so it's foamy and tasty.

Pedia Sure, Nutra/Shakes, Great Shake, and Recovery Power Foods can all be used as between-meal snacks or as complete meals. It seems appropriate to use them as mini-meals, as a beverage at mealtime, or as a snack before bedtime.

## Medicinal-Supplemental Foods to Rest an Angry Gut

During a flare-up, physicians usually recommend that people stop eating to rest their digestive system and rely on predigested food. During the period following the flare-up, after the gut's anger has subsided, some people continue to live on liquids. Medicinal-supplemental foods can help you get through this period.

Jell-O and clear broth give you something for your mouth and stomach, but little nutrition, unless the broth is made especially for the purpose. Indeed, a broth is likely to do more harm than good if its electrolyte balance is off. This is often the case with bouillon, beef consommé, and processed chicken soup, which are usually loaded with sodium and lack potassium. Jell-O is the poorest-quality protein available in the food store! On a protein quality scale, gelatin protein registers too low to sustain life, and when your diet is limited, it can do more harm than good. Use Jell-O as a dessert, but not for nutrition.

Certain foods made for complete nutrition are low residue and can provide complete vitamin-mineral nutrition in 1,000 calories. You can double up on them and get 2,000 calories. Better still, you can add flax oil to them for even better caloric nutrition. Other products, such as the Enteral Nutritional Products made by Mead Johnson, require 2,000 calories to provide the same complete nutrition. A review of a few of these products will illustrate how effectively they can be used.

*Sustacal Liquid* is a liquid food supplement that provides 25 percent of the RDI in a large glassful (8 fluid ounces). It's lactose and fiber free and routinely used for extra nutrition by athletes, pregnant women, and preoperative and postoperative patients. In short, it's designed for people who need high-quality nutrition with no residue and no lactose.

*Sustacal Powder* can be mixed with milk, water, or soy beverage. Mixed with water it delivers more than 25 percent of the RDI for all the important nutrients (less vitamins D, $B_2$ and $B_{12}$) and has a K-factor of just about 3. If mixed with milk or soy beverage, it delivers more nutrition because you get added nourishment. I prefer soy to help eliminate animal fat and increase the omega-3 oils.

*Sustacal Pudding* gives you some variety; 250 calories provides 15 percent of the U.S. RDI in protein, vitamins, and minerals, with a K-factor of just about 3. An added advantage of these foods is their fat distribution, which is about 21 percent of calories as fat, but with an excellent proportion of polyunsaturated, monounsaturated, and saturated fat. Obviously these products have been designed for nutrition.

*Sustacal with Fiber* is the same nutritionally complete product as regular Sustacal, with 1.4 grams of additional dietary fiber in one 250-calorie serving. Suppose you're recovering from a flare-up and have been using Sustacal Liquid and a limited amount of low-fiber food, or no food at all; using Sustacal with Fiber is an excellent way to start introducing dietary fiber slowly without the consequences that might develop from eating regular food. To add extra fiber, Metamucil is the first choice because it has been tested with IBD patients.

*Ensure Liquid* is a liquid food supplement that provides 100 percent of the RDI for all nutrients in 2,000 calories in eight 8-ounce servings. It delivers high-quality, lactose- and fiber-free nutrition, and is ideal for people who can drink liquids, but should have no residue and no lactose.

*Enrich* provides the same nutrient delivery and contains 3.4 grams of dietary fiber in 250 calories; that's 8 ounces. In 2,000 calories, it will deliver 100 percent of the RDI and about 13 grams of dietary fiber. This is an excellent choice once your flare-up has subsided and you can introduce fiber once again.

## Criticare HN, Vital HN: Food That's Predigested

There's one last step before total parenteral nutrition: products such as *Criticare HN* or *Vital HN* supply predigested protein in a ready-to-use liquid. These products permit the digestive system to relax while providing complete nutrition.

"Predigested protein" means the protein has already been broken down into small units that can be absorbed without digestion by your own enzymes. These products also have high levels of vitamins and minerals that compensate for malabsorption.

*Criticare* provides 72 grams of predigested protein in 2,000 calories, together with 100 percent of the RDI for all vitamins, minerals, and electrolytes. Only 3 percent of its calories are derived from fat that has been carefully selected from safflower oil. This means it also provides the essential oils and linoleic and linolenic acids. Criticare is an excellent product capable of sustaining life indefinitely.

*Vital* provides 42 grams of predigested protein in 1,500 calories and 100 percent of the RDI for vitamins and minerals. Therefore, if you're on a predigested diet of 2,000 calories, you'd get about 56 grams of predigested protein and more than 130 percent of the RDI for vitamins and minerals.

Vital is available as a dry powder that is mixed with water. This makes for convenient storage, rapid preparation—and the vanilla flavor is quite pleasant.

Criticare or Vital should be used on the recommendation of a physician and dietitian, or if you feel you need nutritional support. Both come in 8-ounce bottles that make them convenient to store and to use. Whenever food is out of the question and you're told to use clear liquid, ask the doctor if you can try either of these products. You'll be getting sound nutrition that requires the minimum participation of your digestive system.

## Medicinal-Supplemental Foods as a Total Diet

No one wants to live exclusively on a liquid diet, but people have been sustained on these foods for months and have thrived. While it is not the most pleasant way to obtain nourishment, it works quite well when necessary.

# TABLE 8.1

## Supplemental Food Products

| Product | Comments | Corporation |
| --- | --- | --- |
| *Products Made with Milk* | | |
| Great Shake | Ready to drink<br>Concentrated<br>240 calories/6 oz | Menu Magic<br>1717 West 10th St.<br>Indianapolis, IN 46222<br>800-732-5805<br>317-635-9500 |
| Nutra/Shakes | Ready to drink | Nutra/Balance Prod.<br>　Corp.<br>800-432-3134 |
| Recovery Power<br>Foods | Mix in cold water<br>300 calories<br>Excellent fat balance | Great Circles Inc.<br>P.O. Box 1250<br>Montpelier, VT 05601<br>800-872-0611 |
| *Lactose-free Products* | | |
| Sustacal Liquid | Convenient<br>Ready to use | Mead Johnson Corp.<br>Evansville, IN 47721<br>800-247-7893 |
| Sustacal Mix | Made with<br>milk (Lactaid)<br>or water | Mead Johnson Corp. |
| Sustacal with Fiber | Convenient<br>1.4 grams fiber per<br>8 oz (750 calories) | Mead Johnson Corp. |
| Ensure Liquid | Convenient<br>Ready to use | Ross Laboratories<br>Columbus, OH 43216 |
| Ensure Plus | Extra calories<br>Excellent fat balance<br>No fiber | Ross Laboratories |
| Ensure with Fiber | Convenient<br>3.4 grams fiber per 8 fl oz | Ross Laboratories |

| Product | Comments | Corporation |
|---------|----------|-------------|

### *High-Protein Predigested Products*

| Product | Comments | Corporation |
|---------|----------|-------------|
| Criticare HN | High nitrogen elemental diet Ready to use Predigested protein | Bristol-Myers Co. Evansville, IN 47721 800-892-9201 |
| Vital HN | High nitrogen elemental diet Mix with water Predigested protein | Ross Laboratories Columbus, OH 43216 |

# PART II

## Dietary Management of Inflammation: Taming a Bad Gut

Every person who has some form of IBD hopes it will just disappear so he or she won't have to deal any longer with flare-ups, diarrhea, pain, bloody stools, or the social problems that come with these symptoms. Indeed, I have met gregarious people whose social lives are crippled by Crohn's disease. Research indicates that diet can make a tremendous difference in these people's lives and also help medication work much more effectively.

Scientists have proven that modifying the diet to reduce inflammation achieves three major objectives:

- Inflammation is reduced, so flare-ups are less frequent.
- Tissue damage is reduced.
- Flare-ups are less devastating.

In short, the "angry gut" is tamed. So, by following this dietary approach in conjunction with the newer drugs, you have a winning combination.

This section provides a short lesson on inflammation and the tissue damage that accompanies it. You will gain new insights into the nutritional challenges that IBD creates:

- How diet and sensible supplements work together.
- How the new drugs work.
- And why diet and sensible supplements make them more effective.

Finally, all the information is put together in a plan that helps you choose your snacks, meals, supplements, and even your lifestyle.

# CHAPTER 9

# *People Who Don't Get Inflammatory Diseases*

Every ethnic and cultural diet and lifestyle pattern is actually a field experiment in nutrition. And when scientists can compare two groups with similar genetic backgrounds but markedly different food patterns, they can uncover dietary influences on health. Computers have helped make these dietary comparisons possible because they allow scientists to process and compare enormous amounts of information about large numbers of people who live in diverse locations, while matching them by age, height, weight, and any other pertinent factors. These studies let scientists view cultural differences as if they were ongoing experiments in nutrition.

Scientists who conduct these population studies are called epidemiologists; I like to call them "medical detectives." Their major objective is to discover why an illness is prevalent in one population and not in another. Epidemiologists have discovered the causes of cancer; the relationship of salt, weight, and other factors in high blood pressure; the relevance of fat to heart disease; and on the lighter side, that a glass of red wine daily helps you live longer by reducing heart disease. Modern medicine owes much to "medical detectives," because they establish differences upon which future research is based.

Another use for these scientific findings is in guiding public health. It's an important service to make people aware of the connection between such things as lung cancer and smoking, antioxidants and cancer prevention, and saturated fat and heart disease. Less publicly noteworthy, but especially important to you, is that they have uncovered the clues to both prevention and dietary modulation of inflammatory diseases in general, and rheumatoid arthritis and inflammatory bowel disease (IBD) in particular.

## Comparing Greenlanders to Danes

In 1980, a Scandinavian medical journal published a study that compared Greenlanders to their counterparts in Denmark. Comparing Greenlanders to Danes was no coincidence. They have the same Nordic background with similar genetic makeup, and they form what is called a "homogeneous" population. Over the centuries, their diets have remained similar in levels of fat, but are very different in fat composition. Scientists wanted to learn if the differences in the types of fat eaten had an impact on health. Other dietary components, such as carbohydrates and protein, weren't significantly different, which is one more reason the comparison was so important. The senior scientist in this study, Dr. Jorn Dyerberg, emphasized the low heart-disease rate among Greenlanders even though their diet contained as much or more fat than diets in most Western countries—including Denmark. This discovery was important because heart disease is the most expensive health problem facing any country. However, along with heart disease, the scientists looked into statistics regarding inflammatory diseases. Their findings were startling.

## Table 9.1

### Relative Health Differences Between Danes and Greenlanders

| Disease | Incidence Among Danes | Incidence Among Greenlanders |
|---|---|---|
| Heart attack | XXXXX | X |
| Stroke | XX | XXXX |
| Psoriasis | XXXXX | X |
| Diabetes | XXXXX | None |
| Asthma | XXXXX | None |
| Thyroid toxicosis | XXXXX | X |
| Multiple sclerosis | XXXXX | None |
| Epilepsy | X | XX |
| Rheumatoid arthritis | XXXXX | X |
| Ulcers | XXXXX | XX |
| Cancer | XXXXX | XXX |
| Breast cancer | XXXXX | None |
| Inflammatory bowel disease | XXXX | None |

X: a measurable level but very small.
XX: definite and consistent signs of the disease.
XXX: average occurrence of the disease.
XXXX: high incidence of the disease.
XXXXX: very high incidence of the disease.

Inflammatory diseases, especially rheumatoid arthritis, were low among Greenlanders, and IBD simply didn't exist. Besides IBD and rheumatoid arthritis, the other autoimmune, inflammatory diseases included psoriasis, asthma, and multiple sclerosis, which were so low as to be nonsignificant. Though the findings on inflammatory disease were unexpected from a public health standpoint, they paled in comparison to those regarding heart disease and some types of cancer. Although publicity in the news media surrounding these studies focused on cancer and heart disease, scientists asked: "What protected Greenlanders from IBD? From rheumatoid arthritis?" The answer lies in the difference between omega-3 and omega-6 oils.

# A Glossary of Ten Terms About Fat

Although I will repeat often the differences between the omega-3 and omega-6 oils, this glossary can help you with terms used in this book. People who don't work with these terms daily, including scientists, tend to get them mixed up. I find these ten terms help me and my colleagues keep them straight. You might also find them helpful.

| Fat | Abbreviation | What It Is |
| --- | --- | --- |
| 1. Fat | None | A food substance that provides 9 calories per gram or 252 per ounce. |
| 2. Hard Fat | None | A fat that is hard at room temperature, such as the "white" fat around beef, or butter. |
| 3. Oil | None | A fat in liquid form at room temperature that provides 9 calories per gram. |
| 4. Fatty Acid | FA | The smallest unit of all fats (and oils). The term *acid* refers to their structure. |
| 5. Saturated Fat or Saturated Fatty Acid | SFA | A fat consisting of fatty acids that have no open (unsaturated) regions. Usually solid at room temperature. |
| 6. Monounsaturated Fatty Acid | MFA | An oil with one open (unsaturated)area on its fatty acids. Heavy liquid at room temperature, such as olive oil. |
| 7. Polyunsaturated Fat or Polyunsaturated Fatty Acid | PUFA | An oil with many open (unsaturated) areas on its fatty acids. Light in color and liquid at room temperature. The more unsaturated, the lighter the liquid. |
| 8. Omega-3 Oil or Omega-3 PUFA | O-3 | A PUFA in which the unsaturated areas are in a unique location: the third bond from the omega end. |

| Fat | Abbreviation | What It Is |
|---|---|---|
| 9. Omega-6 Oil or Omega-6 PUFA | O-6 | A PUFA in which the unsaturated areas are in a unique location: the sixth bond from the omega end. |
| 10. Essential Fatty Acid or Essential Oils | EFA | PUFAs that are essential for human health, if not life itself. We must get some O-3 and O-6 oils in our diet. |

## Dietary Differences in Greenlanders and Danes

Table 9.2 tells us a great deal about the dietary differences between Greenlanders and Danes.

### Table 9.2

### Dietary Fat Composition

| Dietary Fat | Danes | Greenlanders |
|---|---|---|
| Percentage of calories from fat | 42 | 39 |
| Percentage of saturated fat | 53 | 23 |
| Percentage of monounsaturated fat | 34 | 58 |
| Percentage of polyunsaturated fat | 13 | 19 |
| Total cholesterol, in milligrams | 420 | 700 |
| Ratio of polyunsaturated to saturated fat | 0.2 | 0.8 |

#### Polyunsaturated Fat Intake

| | Danes | Greenlanders |
|---|---|---|
| Omega-3, in grams | 3 | 14 |
| Omega-6, in grams | 10 | 5 |
| Ratio of omega-6 to omega-3 | 3.3 | 0.4 |
| Ratio of omega-3 to omega-6 | 0.3 | 2.8 |

Let's review the features one at a time.

- At 39 and 42 percent, both diets are excessive in fat. These fat levels are similar to those seen in European and North American countries and are becoming common among affluent Asians. It's the result of fast living and fast food, and a shift from their traditional diets.

- Greenlanders eat a diet much more abundant in unsaturated oils (77 percent) compared to Danes (47 percent). The ratio of polyunsaturated to saturated fat makes this difference more obvious.

- Greenlanders eat much more omega-3 oils (14 grams daily) than the Danes (at most, 3 grams daily), making the ratio of omega-3 oils to omega-6 oils about a tenfold difference at 2.8 versus 0.3. The importance of these differences will be discussed later. This difference in the omega-3 and omega-6 oils explains the difference in the disease patterns in Table 9.1, because omega-3 and omega-6 oils have a distinctly different effect on body functions.

With a few exceptions, people eating a meat-rich diet are in the same or worse situation as the Danes with respect to fat composition. The exceptions are seen in parts of Italy and Greece in the Mediterranean, where there are more monounsaturated oils (MFAs) in the diet, because olive oil is so widely used. People in the seacoast villages of Japan, Canada, and other maritime countries eat more fish than their inland counterparts, and their diets are similarly richer in omega-3 oils and other polyunsaturated oils. However, as overfishing makes fish more expensive, even maritime people switch to meat, and the omega-3 oils are becoming an even smaller part of their diets as well.

If you didn't know about the different oils in the diets of Danes and Greenlanders, you'd expect both of them to have a similarly high rate of heart disease. You might even predict that the Greenlanders would be worse off than the Danes because of their cholesterol intake. Dyerberg and researchers who followed his lead took a careful look at the blood fats of the two groups. After all, diets can be misinterpreted and people can often lie about what they eat, but blood analysis gives a true picture.

By comparing blood and blood-cell composition, scientists learn much about the fat in someone's diet. The fat freely circulating in the blood measures what a person ate recently, while the blood-cell fat—the platelets—measures what he's been eating all along.

As an aside, in my own nutrition research from food studies, I learned that each home houses "four families":

1. What foods they tell you they eat.
2. What their refrigerator, freezer, and cupboard indicate they eat.
3. What their garbage shows they eat.
4. What a thorough blood, urine, and stool analysis proves they eat.

The only definitive proof was what Dyerberg found in the blood and tissue of the Danes and Greenlanders.

## Greenlanders and Danes Are What They Eat

Dyerberg's comparison of Danes and Greenlanders was very revealing. Indeed, in light of subsequent research following these findings, it tells us why there was no inflammatory disease in Greenlanders (or other people who eat lots of fish). Greenlanders eat more fish, which is high in omega-3 fat—and inflammatory disease is rampant in Western societies where people eat less fish, or no fish, and more meat. Table 9.3 compares the blood and platelet fats in the Greenlanders and Danes.

## Table 9.3

### Polyunsaturated Fat Composition of Danes and Greenlanders

| Oil | Danes | | Greenlanders | |
|---|---|---|---|---|
| | Percentage | Ratio* O-6/O-3 | Percentage | Ratio* O-6/O-3 |
| *Blood Fat* | | | | |
| Omega-6** | 30.7 | | 8.0 | |
| | | 7.7 | | 0.7 |
| Omega-3*** | 4.0 | | 11.0 | |
| *Platelets (Tissue Fat)* | | | | |
| Omega-6** | 30.3 | | 12.4 | |
| | | 15.2 | | 0.9 |
| Omega-3*** | 2.0 | | 13.8 | |

*The omega-6 total divided by the omega-3 total.
**Omega-6 figure is the sum of linoleic acid and arachidonic acid (AA).
***Omega-3 figure is the sum of EPA and DHA.

Let's analyze the data in Table 9.3.

- Freely circulating blood fat and tissue fat (platelets) were remarkably different in Danes and Greenlanders. Both blood and tissue fat indicate that the Danes eat a diet high in omega-6 oils and the Greenlanders eat a diet rich in omega-3 oils. This confirms the diet analysis and proves that the axiom "We are what we eat" applies to Greenlanders and Danes.
- The ratio of omega-6 to omega-3 is very important; it is obtained by simply dividing omega-6 by omega-3.
- The platelet ratio shows a striking difference. In Chapter Twenty you will learn that these ratios are a telling difference because there is a type of competition that takes place between these oils that either favors or prevents inflammation. The ratio tells us that if an omega-3

oil must compete against an omega-6 oil, it would have an advantage in the Greenlander's body, but about a 15 to 1 disadvantage in the Dane's diet. In short, the Danes have a nominal 15 to 1 disadvantage regarding arthritis and other inflammatory diseases while the Greenlanders have an advantage!

## Faeroe Islanders Versus Danes

The eighteen Faeroe Islands located in the North Atlantic are self-ruled, but they have elected representatives in the Danish parliament and are part of the same genetic pool. Comparing them to Danes is like comparing Greenlanders to Danes. The results are very similar, if not identical.

The comparison of inflammatory and heart disease rates among the Faeroe Islanders and among the Danes is identical to the Greenlander-Dane comparison. Inflammatory diseases in the islanders are a fraction of those seen in the Danes, and IBD *doesn't exist,* even though the dietary comparisons are the same.

## Japanese Inlanders Versus Seacoast Inhabitants

Japan probably has the world's most homogeneous population. With very little immigration and centuries of relative isolation, it's safe to conclude that comparing seacoast Japanese to inland villagers eliminates any genetic variations, and the differences observed will have to do with diet and lifestyle. Sure enough, scientists observe the same difference between Japanese seacoast villagers and inland villagers as are seen between Greenlanders and Danes. Even skeptics must take notice.

Since the original studies comparing Danes to Greenlanders, scientists have sought out comparisons where there are reasonably similar ethnic backgrounds with different dietary and lifestyle characteristics. Hence, we have learned the following:

- Canadians in maritime provinces, where cold-water fish is a dietary staple, have much less inflammatory diseases in general.
- Italians who live inland and eat a diet rich in meat have more inflammatory disease than those who live on the seacoast and eat fish.
- Asians who migrate to the United States and take on our meat-oriented diet have more inflammatory disease than siblings who remain in Asia and eat a more vegetarian and fish-oriented diet.
- Japanese who live in seacoast villages and eat a diet rich in fish and almost completely exclude meat have much less inflammatory disease than inland villagers who eat meat.
- The most recent research indicates these same patterns hold for multiple sclerosis, which is also an inflammatory autoimmune disease with many similarities to all inflammatory diseases.

These comparisons bear the same findings about inflammatory disease as originally seen in the Dyerberg studies. The magnitude of the differences was not always the same, but the trends were consistent: diet matters.


## Consistent Trends Are Important

When parents boast to grandparents that a young child can talk, silence reigns. However, the grandparents catch snatches of speech here and there, and they perceive a trend and know that their grandchild can speak.

Consistent trends in nutrition and health are more important than specific occurrences because a trend indicates a general direction and rules out any chance occurrence. For example, if an illness consistently declines as a dietary change occurs in a population group that remains the same by other criteria, it discloses a direction that transcends any single event. When scientists observe similar disease trends across other boundaries, such as countries, ethnic groups, latitude, and so on, their findings are much stronger.

## What Dietary Differences Account for These Findings?

Diet is the main difference in all the population studies. More precisely, it's the difference between omega-3 and omega-6 polyunsaturated fats in the diet. So, we need to start by becoming familiar with fats and oils.

Fat is nature's most concentrated energy source. Those Danes studied consumed 42 percent of total calories as fat, and the Greenlanders 39 percent; that is, both Danes and Greenlanders got about 40 percent of their energy from fat. This dietary composition is consistent with that of Europeans, North Americans (Americans, Canadians, and Mexicans), the British, the Faeroe Islanders, and other populations. Scientists generally recognize that dietary fat energy between 39 and 42 percent is not a large difference. For example, once the diet exceeds 30 to 35 percent of calories from fat, heart disease and cancer patterns don't increase. To bring about a change in heart disease and cancer rates, the diet must be below about 25 percent of calories from fat, if general activity patterns are similar. Indeed, until Dr. Dyerberg's findings, it was taken for granted that all such fat levels would have the same disease patterns. How wrong they were.

Greenlanders eat a somewhat unusual diet because it contains the meat of marine mammals, such as walrus, sea lions, and whales. Faeroe Islanders eat fish more than mammals, and Japanese seacoasters and Canadian maritime and arctic groups eat only cold-water fish. These eating patterns hold the key to the differences in their disease rates.

Cold-water fish such as salmon and marine mammals such as sea lions have fats—actually oils—that are markedly different from those we obtain from beef and other domesticated animals. Although it's dangerous to put "logic" into nature's choice, I'll give it a try. Fish take on the water temperature where they live, in contrast to warm-blooded animals, which have a constant body temperature. As you know, animal fat is hard and inflexible at room temperature, let alone at temperatures of 50 degrees Fahrenheit or lower. So eating experience tells you that the fats in these fish are different, and a biochemical analysis confirms your taste. There seems to be some logic in nature's choice: cold-water fish couldn't move in cold water if they had "warm temperature" fat as do animals. Indeed, the fish would be like solid blocks!

Greenlanders, Faeroe Islanders, Japanese seacoasters, and so on eat a diet rich in omega-3 oils (from fish), while most of the world eats a diet rich in omega-6 oils (from meat). The difference was observed in the blood of the Danes and Greenlanders.

As you'll soon learn, one specific omega-6 oil from meat favors inflammation and joint damage, while omega-3 oils suppress inflammation and joint damage. These effects on inflammation aren't direct like medicine; rather, they go through elaborate processes that have only been understood in recent years.

## Fish Is Special

Fish has always had a special place in Christian and Eastern religions; so much so that fasting often permits the consumption of fish. The allowance of fish during fasts seems to predate written dietary rules.

Folk wisdom teaches that fish is brain food. Although this belief is similarly enmeshed in antiquity, it was revived in the 1920s when scientists discovered that fish contained phosphorus, which they felt provided mental energy. They were wrong; phosphorus isn't the essential element involved in this function, but it didn't take long for biochemists to learn that the essential omega-3 fish oils do find their way into the human brain and are critical for mental function, intelligence level (to some extent), and behavior.

Although brain food doesn't *seem* related to IBD, there is a definite link.

Comparisons among vegans (who eat no animal products whatsoever), lacto-ovo vegetarians (who eat dairy products and eggs), and fish-eating vegetarians show they all have lower levels of inflammatory disease when compared with omnivores (people who eat everything). But even more exciting is that vegans and fish-eating vegetarians have the lowest levels of this disease when compared with omnivores.

In addition, vegetarians get omega-3 oils from numerous vegetables (especially leafy varieties) and from nuts and seeds (such as walnuts, almonds, pecans, and flaxseed) that are rich in omega-3 oils. A vegetarian's diet is usually much lower in fat than a meat eater's diet. Therefore, the correct oils (omega-3), though not as abundant in their diet, don't have as much competition with omega-6 oils. More important for our discussion, these diets are also devoid of the one oil—arachidonic acid—which, we'll see in Chapter Twenty, is critical in causing inflammation.

Vegetarians, especially vegans, have one more thing going for them. A low-fat, nonmeat diet seems to reduce inflammation and flare-ups in general. This result derives from two sources: (1) red meat seems to aggravate inflammatory disease and (2) the correct dietary fiber, which only comes from vegetables, definitely helps relieve inflammation.

> The vegetarian diet that permits fish is just about the ideal diet for people with inflammatory diseases.

In Chapter Eleven we'll discuss studies in which scientists applied this observation in a clinical environment with excellent results. In addition, fish oil capsules and flax oil (a vegetarian source of EPA) produced good results.

# CHAPTER 10

# The Basis of Inflammation and Tissue Damage

Your body has the ability to make substances called prostaglandins that are either "bad" because they increase inflammation, or "good" because they suppress it. Along with each prostaglandin, your body also makes another substance, a leukotriene. If the "bad" prostaglandin aggravates inflammation, the leukotriene causes tissue damage; if the "good" prostaglandin modulates inflammation, the corresponding leukotriene will not aggravate the tissues or cause tissue damage.

Controlling inflammation and damage by diet requires selecting foods and using supplements that suppress the bad prostaglandins and leukotrienes and increase the good ones. Most anti-inflammatory drugs suppress both the bad and good prostaglandins but not the leukotrienes, so even if you take a drug that stops inflammation, tissue damage can continue. However, a new drug recently introduced, Infliximab, moves a step closer to also suppressing tissue damage.

## Metabolism

Your body is the most complex chemical-processing plant you'll ever see, let alone control. Though not as big as an oil refinery, a food plant, or a space shuttle, it's so much more complex, there's no contest.

In a few hours your body can convert a tuna sandwich into body tissues ranging from fingernails (all protein) to muscles (protein, fat, and carbohydrate) to subtle hormones. It can extract the chemical energy locked in fat and sugar more efficiently than your automobile can extract the chemical energy in gasoline or alcohol, which is very similar to fat and carbohydrate. Feel the heat of an automobile engine after it's been running, and notice that it's very much hotter than your body; your body is carrying on the same energy-extraction processes more effectively.

Your car uses just one chemical process—it burns gasoline (similar to fat, sugar, and alcohol) to produce carbon dioxide and water while using the energy to power the car. Your body pulls more energy from the same amount of fuel, does it at body temperature, and keeps at least 25,000 other, infinitely more complicated processes going on at the same time—and all the while you don't even notice. For example, while you burn fuel, you also may be reading a book, the print images of which are converted by chemical processes in our eyes into other chemicals that are passed along a nerve as electrical impulses to your brain, which converts these impulses into the information that you see on the page, and stores it as chemicals in your brain to be recalled in some future instant. If that's not marvelous, tell me what is! And that's just a small fraction of what metabolism accomplishes every instant of your life.

Metabolism is really the sum of two parts. The first is the breaking down of complex substances (tuna sandwich) into basic components, such as fats, proteins, sugars, vitamins, minerals, and a myriad of other substances. The second is the use of these basic substances to build complex substances (muscles, eyes, the memory-storage chemicals in your brain) or to ultimately break them down into carbon dioxide and water for obtaining the energy used for living. Through metabolism, your body extracts substances from food and makes the material it needs to thrive.

# Is Metabolism Magic? No!
# It's All in the Enzymes

Metabolism seemed like magic just a hundred years ago, but now we know it involves the same basic physical laws at work that govern our universe. It's all made possible by an infinite variety of very complex proteins called enzymes, which catalyze the chemical reactions that convert complex things into simple substances and extract energy from them that is used to build complex substances. To "catalyze" means to "bring about change without being changed." You could compare it to the official at a marriage ceremony. Two people are brought together for a ritual that initiates their new and marvelous life together; the official who performs the ritual says a few words, perhaps adds a blessing; when it's over, his or her life goes on as usual, while the individuals who got married will never be the same.

Enzymes are very complex proteins that perform their function at body temperature and, like the wedding official, they remain unchanged when the job is done and cannot change the direction in which the process goes. That's up to physical laws that factor in "need," which is dictated by the final product and the availability of raw materials. While these physical laws (thermodynamics) determine the direction of metabolism, they don't dictate its speed, or the details of the processes involved.

How your body makes prostaglandins and leukotrienes is a good example of metabolism at work. Your body produces either prostaglandin PGE-2 or PGE-3, depending on the fatty acid available (either arachidonic acid [AA] or eicosapentaenoic acid [EPA]). If AA is in large quantity, PGE-2 is produced; if enough EPA is available, PGE-3 is made. However, your body cannot take either prostaglandin and work backward to make fatty acid, so the direction is set by other factors.

## Making Prostaglandins and Leukotrienes

One enzyme group, named cyclooxygenase, can use two oils to make either the good prostaglandin (PGE-3) and its good leukotriene, or the bad prostaglandin (PGE-2) and its similarly bad leukotriene. When the fatty acid eicosapentaenoic acid (EPA) is abundant, your body produces good prostaglandins and leukotrienes that do not cause inflammation; when arachidonic acid (AA) is in large quantity, the bad prostaglandins and leukotrienes are produced, which cause inflammation. Leukotrienes are required for other body processes, so when a prostaglandin is made, a leukotriene is always made at the same time. The body requires both the prostaglandins and leukotrienes to function correctly. Even what we call the bad prostaglandin is necessary in very limited amounts, so it's not all bad outside the context of inflammatory disease. However, the amounts of each prostaglandin produced depend almost completely on the amount of each building material. That's where the omega-3 oil, EPA, and/or the omega-6 oil, AA, enter the story.

This process is illustrated by the following metabolic flow chart, which shows the process much as a road map charts a route. Even though I have oversimplified this chart, it requires careful attention.

## FIGURE 10.1

### The Metabolic Basis of Intestinal Inflammation, Tissue Damage, and Relief Through Diet and Supplementation

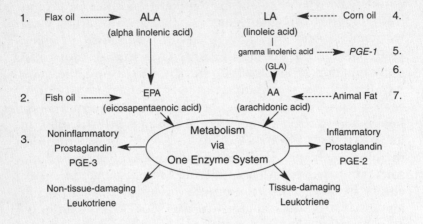

## The Biochemical Basis of Preventing an Inflamed (Angry) Intestine

This metabolic flow chart illustrates how correct food and food-supplement selection can change metabolism to stop intestinal inflammation and damage. The objective of the diet is to reduce production of prostaglandin PGE-2 to the minimum necessary for its essential functions, and to increase production of prostaglandin PGE-3, which does not cause inflammation; similarly for the two corresponding leukotrienes. These changes can be accomplished by sensible food and food-supplement selection.

Each item on this chart is discussed in detail to help you understand how easily it can be put into everyday practice with food and food supplements.

Let's take it a step at a time, starting on the left side of the flow chart:

## 1. ALA (Alpha Linolenic Acid)

ALA is made in the chloroplasts of green plants from another polyunsaturated fatty acid called linoleic acid (shown on the right of the chart). Animals, including humans, can't do this; they can only convert linoleic acid, through a series of steps, into arachidonic acid (AA), which is used to make the antagonistic prostaglandins. ALA is found in all green plants, including green vegetables, leaves, grass, algae, and seaweed. Mammals, including humans, do not manufacture ALA.

ALA has some special positive effects on IBD and general health besides its metabolic conversion to EPA. In studies on its ability as a metabolic material to suppress inflammation through this conversion, an improvement in intestinal absorption was observed. Since this has been observed in both clinical research with human volunteers and in animal studies, there is little doubt of a beneficial effect.

## 2. ALA to EPA

ALA is important because it is converted to EPA. Fish, algae, plankton, and mammals, including man, convert ALA to EPA through normal metabolism. Fish and sea mammals (whales, sea lions, etc.) eat the algae and plankton of the sea, accumulating EPA in their oily tissue. We either eat fish and get EPA or, thanks to technology, remove it from the fish and put it in capsules.

Long ago we consumed animals such as deer, rabbits, and range animals (e.g., buffalo and range-fed cattle) and obtained EPA that accumulated in the muscle tissues of these animals. Still, you don't get nearly as much EPA from range animals as you do from fish. Fish and sea mammals are the richest sources of EPA because many of them live exclusively on plankton or eat other fish that do. Furthermore, fish also produce more EPA to survive in cold ocean temperatures.

## 3. EPA to PGE-3

EPA is converted to the prostaglandin PGE-3. Not all EPA becomes prostaglandin PGE-3; some is made into another essential oil—docosahexaenoic acid (DHA). Read the label on a bottle of EPA capsules carefully, and you will notice they contain some DHA, which helps the diet because a larger portion of EPA can then be made into prostaglandin PGE-3.

A word about DHA is appropriate even if our focus is on EPA and prostaglandin PGE-3. Docosahexaenoic acid is found in all nerve tissue, including our brain and eyes, where research has proven it is absolutely essential. In young children, it has even been proven to have a role in behavior and intelligence. Preliminary research suggests its deficiency in the diet during pregnancy could account for the increase in attention deficit disorder and attention deficit hyperactive disorder. This is one more reason why this diet program has benefits beyond IBD and helps all family members.

**EPA is king of inflammation relief.** EPA is the critical omega-3 fatty acid pertaining to inflammation since it's the only material our bodies use to make the beneficial prostaglandins and leukotrienes that prevent inflammation and tissue damage. Most experts (who have used up to 18 grams of EPA daily in clinical studies) seem to agree that if you eat a diet low in arachidonic acid (found in animal fat), 3 or more grams of EPA per day from fish and supplements should be adequate, and more is fine.

EPA capsules also contain ALA and DHA, an important combination for another reason—the "push-pull" of metabolism. EPA in the presence of adequate DHA is converted to the beneficial prostaglandins. Although your metabolic machinery (look at the metabolic chart again) will not reverse itself to convert EPA to ALA, having some ALA helps drive EPA to the prostaglandin. Sufficient DHA in the capsule leaves no further need for DHA by the body, and all the EPA is used to make the beneficial prostaglandins or is accumulated in other tissues as required. EPA is also found in the blood, the blood cells, and the walls of blood vessels, where it helps to reduce heart disease. Although I'm getting a little far afield, it's another reason why this diet is so healthy—a side effect is that it helps prevent heart disease, stroke, and cancer. So, if everyone in the family follows this plan, they'll be better and more healthy for the effort.

## 4. Linoleic Acid

Linoleic acid is an essential fatty acid from which your body can make all the omega-6 fatty acids it requires. Since most cooking oils and margarines are made from corn oil, or other PUFA oils, most diets provide an abundance, if not an excess, of linoleic acid.

## 5. Linoleic Acid (LA) to Gamma Linolenic Acid (GLA)

Linoleic acid is converted to many other fatty acids, including a transitory, short-lived material called gamma linolenic acid (GLA), another omega-6 oil. By "transitory" and "short-lived," I mean that GLA is not available in quantity because it is used about as quickly as it is made. However, in the presence of an abundance of arachidonic acid (AA), very little, if any, is made. GLA isn't made because an abundance of AA causes "feedback inhibition." This simply means that there is no need for the body to make AA, so the LA to AA system simply shuts down. If you've ever been in a traffic jam, you've got the picture.

## 6. Gamma Linolenic Acid (GLA) and Prostaglandin PGE-1

We get very little GLA in our diets, as it is a seed oil only found most abundantly in evening primrose, or borage, and black currant seeds, which are no longer dietary components. Metabolism converts some GLA to prostaglandin PGE-1. Most researchers recognize that PGE-1 modulates the inflammation caused by PGE-2 when AA is available in modest quantities. Your body can only produce PGE-1 in very minor quantities; consequently, when dietary AA is abundant, the body produces excessive PGE-2, and any beneficial effect of PGE-1 is lost.

However, if you follow the diet and supplement plan explained in this book, your body will produce enough PGE-1 to modulate the inflammatory effects of the small amount of PGE-2 that your tissues will produce. This is one benefit that diet can produce and that no medication yet known, or likely to be developed in the next decade, will offer. So even if we can't stop 100 percent of inflammation, the residual can be modulated by the body's natural metabolism. You simply have to supply the correct starting material.

### 7. Gamma Linolenic Acid (GLA) to Arachidonic Acid (AA)

GLA is generally considered an "intermediate" between linoleic acid (LA) and AA. Our body needs: (1) both GLA and LA, (2) some AA, and (3) the prostaglandin PGE-2. However, when the diet provides excess AA, too much PGE-2 is produced, and the AA swamps the small amount of EPA that is converted by the same enzyme system. A diet rich in AA also renders the small amount of prostaglandin PGE-1 useless.

One more time: A diet rich in animal foods and baked goods made with animal fat (e.g., butter and omega-6 oils) is excessive in arachidonic acid and favors inflammation. The foods and food supplements you select give you complete control over this cycle.

## The Enzymes Aren't Perfect

A serious problem pops up in your metabolism of linoleic acid. Specifically, your body seems equipped to work best in a food environment that is abundant in the omega-3 oils, including ALA and EPA, with limited amounts of the omega-6 oils, LA and especially AA. Since the body expects an abundance of the omega-3 oils, the enzyme system works better with the omega-6 oils, which are expected to be scarce. Our dietary habits have completely turned that system upside down, because we eat foods generally rich in the omega-6 oils and totally lacking in the omega-3 oils. For many people this is not a problem, but it's a metabolic disaster for people with any inflammatory disease.

## Stopping Intestinal and Bowel Inflammation and Tissue Damage

The metabolic flow chart illustrates how correct food and food-supplement selection can change metabolism to stop inflammation and tissue damage. The following six steps are essential in controlling inflammation and damage:

1. Eliminate animal foods—arachidonic acid. This will normalize prostaglandin PGE-2 production.
2. Obtain dietary EPA by eating cold-water fish as your protein source. This will favor prostaglandin PGE-3.
3. Select cooking and salad oils rich in ALA, such as canola oil, to favor natural EPA production.
4. Use flax oil: add it sensibly to food, such as salads and cereals, to favor natural EPA and prostaglandin PGE-3. *Do not fry or bake with flax oil.* Take 30 grams or more of flax oil in capsules, or add it, in liquid form, to food.
5. Sensible EPA supplementation: take at least 2 grams of EPA daily (9 grams daily is safe).
6. Sensible GLA supplementation: take evening primrose or borage oil supplements (1 gram daily) in moderation to favor prostaglandin PGE-1, which modulates the inflammatory effect of prostaglandin PGE-2.

## A Flaw in the System: EPA Versus AA

Now you can visualize your problem. The enzyme (cyclooxygenase) that catalyzes EPA into the good prostaglandin PGE-3 and the good leukotriene works better (scientists say "has a better affinity") with AA because throughout most of human history AA has been scarce. Look at it as a "natural choice" prejudiced by evolution, as directed by the Creator.

This means that if there is an equal amount of AA and EPA available to the enzyme, it would take AA and make prostaglandin PGE-2, leaving EPA sitting on the sideline. So a diet that supplies a lot of AA and a little EPA is predisposed to make only the bad prostaglandin and leukotriene. Worse yet, the average diet is overly excessive in animal fat or omega-6 oils—so the enzyme never sees EPA, and only prostaglandin PGE-2 is made.

The abundance of AA causes another flaw to emerge—the production of PGE-1 is stopped, as I mentioned already. While PGE-1 can't substitute for PGE-2 or PGE-3, it can help modulate some of the inflammation caused by PGE-2. However, in a diet rich in AA, PGE-1 is not made.

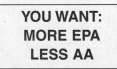

YOU WANT:
MORE EPA
LESS AA

The opposite happens in a diet with more EPA than AA, such as the diets of Greenlanders, seacoast villagers in many countries, and vegetarians. In these diets, the good prostaglandin and leukotriene dominate, because EPA is abundant. However, since the enzyme has a greater affinity for AA, prostaglandin PGE-2 is made in sufficient amounts for its essential functions. Thus, there's no inflammatory disease among people who have a diet rich in EPA. It's not magic, it's simply normal metabolism.

Importantly, in Asian countries and areas where fish and marine life were a dominant, nonvegetarian protein source,

IBD was seldom, if ever, diagnosed. Beginning in the 1950s, meat started becoming a larger part of their diets—a trend that accelerated during the next four decades. Now, as this millennium comes to an end, hamburger and fast-food outlets dominate worldwide. Similarly, IBD, especially Crohn's disease, is growing at an alarming rate. This morbid trend is indirect support for the concepts discussed in this book.

## Why Would the Enzymes Prefer AA?

Your body's enzymes reflect the food environment in which humans developed. Just a few hundred years ago, let alone 1,000 or 10,000 years or more, alpha linolenic acid (ALA), eicosapentaenoic acid (EPA), and docosahexaenoic acid (DHA) were plentiful in the foods our ancestors ate. Salads were made from purslane, a vegetable rich in ALA. Range animals fed on grasses that were rich in ALA, so their meat was limited in arachidonic acid (AA) and rich in ALA, EPA, and DHA; the same was true for rabbits and other small game animals.

In contrast, linoleic acid (LA) was not very abundant, and AA was quite scarce since it's strictly an animal material. After all, for much of our history we were mostly vegetarian, and meat came from game, which contains EPA and AA. Farm animals in those times ate grass and straw, not corn, which was a New World food that was not produced in enough quantity to feed animals. With these omega-3 oils in abundance, the enzyme served our needs well, because AA was scarce in our diets and necessary for the prostaglandin PGE-2. Hence, the fact that the enzyme works more efficiently on AA than it does on EPA only reflects our early environment. By favoring AA, a scarce material was converted to a material needed in limited quantity. This is just another example of the efficiency of the human body and how slowly we change.

This enzyme preference for AA suggests that there is a logic to evolution—that the hand of God favored a more modest diet. Both interpretations are correct. Evolution's logic is survival and the ability to thrive.

Once again, balance plays an important role in the metabolic picture. When PGE-2 is produced in minor quantities, the other prostaglandin PGE-1, similarly produced in limited quantities, seems to balance PGE-2's inflammatory impact. However, PGE-1 is produced in very limited quantities, so a food environment that provides excess AA will never provide enough PGE-1. Worse yet, when dietary AA is available, the production of PGE-1 stops, suggesting a sort of metabolic traffic jam.

## A System Gone Wrong

If you have IBD and your diet favors the wrong foods, you probably take drugs that suppress PGE-3 but also prevent PGE-2 production. So while you diminish the inflammation, you actually cause long-term problems. It's instructive to consider each factor.

First, a diet that has been excessive in animal fat has created fat reserves high in AA. Add to those fat reserves a continuous dietary supply of AA, and the dominant (if not only) prostaglandin produced is PGE-2. Therefore, inflammation is favored, and its accompanying leukotriene continues to favor tissue damage.

Second, while PGE-1 seems to suppress the inflammation caused by PGE-2, it only works in an environment where there is very little PGE-2, not one in which it dominates. To make matters worse, there are no common dietary sources of gamma linolenic acid (GLA) from which PGE-1 is made, so only very small amounts are produced naturally by the body. However, as we saw in Chapter Seven, when GLA is taken as a supplement, it seems to suppress inflammation.

Third, a diet rich in AA cannot possibly supply enough EPA to produce prostaglandin PGE-3. This means the prostaglandin-producing enzyme system will continue making large quantities of PGE-2 and no PGE-3. If that's not bad enough, the use of typical NSAIDs (nonsteroid anti-inflammatory drugs) makes matters worse.

Fourth, when NSAIDs are used in this dietary environment, they suppress the inflammation by stopping PGE-3 and thus bring relief to the victim. But they also precipitate other problems; for while NSAIDs prevent PGE-3, they don't stop leukotriene production. There is one bit of good news, however. Although leukotriene production does cause some tissue damage, it is probably suppressed by the general slowdown of prostaglandin production.

This is where metabolic maps resemble roads. It's as if a bridge is jammed, causing tie-ups in all the peripheral roads so that nothing moves. Sticking with the road map and clogged intersections analogy, we can summarize the following diet design:

- Aggressively minimize dietary AA to stop excess PGE-2.
- Moderate dietary linoleic acid to support natural PGE-2 levels and natural PGE-1.
- Aggressively increase dietary ALA and EPA.
- Use EPA and/or ALA supplements sensibly to favor PGE-3.
- Use GLA supplements sensibly to make PGE-1.
- Make sure your diet plan is abundant in vegetable foods and provides dietary fiber.

If we put these points to work correctly, the dietary program will increase EPA naturally, elevate the good prostaglandins, and diminish the bad prostaglandins, as the clinical studies have verified.

## Why Follow a Diet? Why Not Just Take Omega-3 Oil Supplements?

Clinical studies that focus on omega-3 oil supplements make a diet plan look difficult, if not complex. Make a complete dietary and supplement commitment, and you will get better results than by simply cutting out meat and using omega-3 oil supplements. If you do the latter, you are not likely to ever achieve your maximum potential. In a way, you'd be using a food supplement (omega-3 oils) as if it were a medicine, which it isn't. You've got to eat, so do it correctly and maximize your results. In nutrition, teamwork is essential, and you should optimize everything to get the best results.

In clinical research, volunteers are usually living at home and eating on their own. As a rule, they are given a diet to follow, but the clinical researcher cannot count on it. So the only solution is to give the volunteers large amounts of EPA; in fact, most studies give them from 6 to 9 grams daily, and in some studies as much as 18 grams. Those levels are fine for the study, but unrealistic for the average person with IBD. The researcher's objective is to prove that it works. After the proof, it is up to the individual to make it work in real life on a daily basis.

Diet can accomplish something supplements cannot. Glance again at Figure 10.1 and recognize that eicosapentaenoic acid (EPA) competes with arachidonic acid (AA) to make either a good or bad prostaglandin. Diet makes that competition work in your favor by minimizing AA and maximizing EPA on a consistent basis. Sensible supplementation with omega-3 oils can make a diet work much better than doing either one alone, but only diet can reduce the level of AA. A dietary approach is holistic, in that it uses all the research findings rather than focusing on a single path.

## Total Body Fat

Now understanding the basis of inflammation, you know that along with changing your diet, there's another approach that will yield significant benefits to optimize your total body fat reserves. Those reserves will always have a complement of AA, and the objective is to bring that level into balance with the omega-3 oils. This will happen naturally if you're consistent with diet, supplements, and exercise.

Yes, exercise is also key to your success. You don't have to become an athlete; you just have to do regular, moderate exercise, such as a brisk walk. Swimming is even better. And you can develop a reasonable alternative with one of the many fat-burning and muscle-building devices. Chapter Twenty-four is devoted to fitness and will cover these options in detail.

## Leukotrienes and Tissue Damage

We focused our attention on the prostaglandins to help you gain a working knowledge of inflammation as a metabolic outcome. Indeed, once you have time to digest all the concepts, you will see how diet and sensible supplements can reduce, if not stop, inflammation. But what about tissue damage?

Production of the leukotrienes are in proportion to the prostaglandins. However, leukotrienes should be looked upon as the tip of an iceberg. In contrast to the prostaglandins, leukotrienes are metabolized further to many other materials that cause tissue damage. However, they don't cause the damage directly, but indirectly, by initiating what we call free radical reactions.

These free radicals are complex, short-lived (less than .0001 second) materials that cause tissue damage. While the good prostaglandin and its good leukotriene don't cause the damage, there is always some of the bad leukotriene produced. So the question is: How else can you stop the free radicals?

Since any free radical process is also what chemists call an "oxidative process," the antioxidants are nature's way of stopping them. I like to think of free radicals as nature's explosives, and the antioxidants as nature's antidemolition experts.

Vitamin E is an antioxidant that works best in intestinal tissues. That is why I urge you to take about 400 IU of vitamin E daily. (See page 92 in Chapter Seven.)

## How Drugs Work

Inspect Figure 10.1 and ask yourself how you would control Crohn's disease if you had a magic drug. If you said, "I would reduce prostaglandin PGE-2 so that just enough is produced for vital functions, but not an excess to cause inflammation beyond what PGE-1 can handle," you would be right.

If you had such a drug, you would be able to help people with Crohn's disease, rheumatoid arthritis, multiple sclerosis, psoriasis, probably asthma, and many other illnesses where inflammation is a major factor.

The enzyme system cyclooxygenase is the target of many drugs, beginning with aspirin, the simplest. The newest and most sophisticated drug, Infliximab, is the most specific and targets the enzyme system better than any previous drug. Although it is far from perfect, it brings everything a giant step closer.

The major objective of any drug is to stop unwanted functions, but it inhibits some necessary functions as well. Consequently, all drugs have side effects that fall into two categories: short-term and long-term.

Short-term effects include rash, chest pains, chills, and either low or high blood pressure; all either subside or the patient simply gets used to them.

Long-term side effects usually don't show up until years of regular use. In the case of some drugs, the side effects are well known. However, with new drugs, only time will tell what the long-term effects will be. This is one more reason to pursue a diet that will minimize the amount of medication required and the side effects associated with it. It is an excellent example of teamwork, where you and your physician are partners in optimizing your health.

# CHAPTER 11

# *Clinical Research Results:*
# *Inflammation Can Be Managed*

Research has consistently shown that both inflammation and tissue damage can be suppressed by diet and sensible supplementation. Especially important to IBD patients are the findings that nutrient absorption improves when inflammation is suppressed. Consequently, the IBD patient can and should take an active role in minimizing flare-ups and making them milder when they do occur.

## Clinical Studies Are Necessary

I've explored with you the metabolism that causes or reduces inflammation and explained some scientific observations. This knowledge has been put into a dietary program that could achieve this objective. Up to now, we've studied inflammation through the eyes of biochemists as metabolism. Shouldn't it also be scientifically tested to convince you that theory can be put into practice? This is where clinical studies enter the picture.

No matter how good our knowledge of nutrition, biochemistry, and metabolism, the human body can surprise us with unexpected shifts. That is why scientists do clinical studies—to rule out flaws in their thinking and to uncover the unexpected.

## Double-Blind: Avoiding the Placebo Effect

Any results from a clinical test can be influenced by the attitudes of clinicians, assistants, and patients, not to mention the volunteers with IBD. Scientists call this influence the placebo effect, and it can account for as much as a 15 percent improvement—no matter what's done. In other words, 15 percent of the participants could do significantly better even if you just gave them a starch pill (called a placebo) and lots of encouragement. A placebo is given because scientists recognize that attitude can produce either improvement or failure (although it's usually improvement). Think about research objectives for a moment and you'll get the point.

For example, a researcher reviews scientific findings and develops a hypothesis about the omega-3 oil EPA and IBD relief. The scientist then writes a carefully thought-out research proposal, seeking grant money to test the hypothesis in a clinical study. He or she believes the omega-3 oils will improve IBD and sets out to prove it. With the urgent needs in clinical medicine and competition for scarce resources, researchers can't afford to spend time proving a negative. Hence, research scientists are aiming to prove their ideas, so their attitudes have to be positive.

Second, the IBD volunteer looks to improve his or her life through a new treatment and hopes that the sacrifice he or she makes by being a guinea pig will help other similarly afflicted people. Consequently, positive attitude contributes to a personal desire to get better and to help others.

Now add a close working relationship between the clinician and the patient volunteer, who might see one or more staff members weekly, if not every few days. Enthusiasm is infectious and everyone's spirits lift as they always do around positive people. Add the fact that most people with a chronic illness never get involved in seeking a cure.

It all adds up to a simple point: everyone in the study is pulling hard for good results. If studies aren't carefully designed, about a 15 percent improvement will be observed since the placebo effect is never negative. A well-designed study will rule out the placebo effect, so the outcome of the treatment will be clear.

Double-blind studies eliminate the placebo effect. This safeguard simply ensures that the patients don't know whether they are getting the real thing (in this case, the omega-3 oil) or a placebo. Nor does the researcher know which patient is getting the oil. An accountant or similarly uninvolved person codes the materials, locks the code in a safe, and releases it only after all the results are tabulated by a disassociated statistician. Scientists can then compare results against the actual material used.

## Crossover Studies: Each Person Is a Control

Another approach often used in food-related studies is a crossover design. This variation means each patient will get both the real omega-3 oil and a placebo—at different times in a random order among volunteers. For example, some patients get omega-3 oil for three months while others get a placebo. A "washout" period follows, when all the patients take nothing and follow a similar diet, then the supplements are reversed. Hence, this crossover study is also double-blind, providing comparisons between patients, but it has the added value that each patient acts as his or her own control.

Time is a disadvantage in the crossover design, because it's difficult to keep a study going for six to twelve months. After all, the patients must be able to alter their lives sufficiently so that they can come to the clinic and submit to blood tests and physical evaluations. In addition, the longer the study, the greater its cost, so there's a financial consideration as well. However, it's a superb method, since the crossover design eliminates a variable that has emerged in some IBD studies. EPA creates a somewhat fishy aftertaste in some people because of normal variations in the muscle that closes the stomach. This means that some people will know when they're getting something "fishy." The crossover design is the best way to rule out this guessing game.

## Single-Blind: Dietary Studies Can't Be Double-Blind

A necessary variation in dietary studies is the "single-blind" technique. Face it, a diet that contains fish instead of meat or poultry, or is vegetarian, is obvious to those who do the eating, let alone to people who do the cooking and serving. Indeed, you can even tell whether or not you're eating some variety of fish, rather than beef or turkey. Therefore, scientists use the single-blind approach in most dietary studies.

A single-blind study usually means the patient knows his diet is different even if he's getting a daily pill that is double-blinded. However, even if the patient is aware of the diet, it can still be hidden from the clinician who is evaluating the results. In fact, the clinician can be recruited outside the study as an evaluator and instructed to discuss only physical changes, symptoms (stools, blood levels, etc.), or illness. In this way, single-blind dietary studies are completely objective with no placebo effect.

## IBD's Special Research Challenges

IBD is much more difficult to study than other inflammatory diseases. Your own experience teaches you that the major problems are with the flare-ups. Just think of the following questions:

- If a flare-up occurs during a diet study, should you stick with the diet?
- Should the research scientist use steroids to put your flare-up in remission, and then give EPA or a diet with EPA?
- Should you continue taking steroids or other medication?

- Should the researchers try injecting EPA (or other omega-3 oil) directly into your blood, or into animals in which researchers can create IBD?

As you have probably reasoned, the above variations and combinations of them have all been attempted. In general, the results are quite rewarding and research is continuing.

## Results with IBD

While IBD is not only special and more complicated than rheumatoid arthritis, the results with diet and supplements are generally the same. Taking EPA and flax oil as supplements has not only prolonged remission, but has reduced leukotriene production. Animal studies have been especially rewarding and confirm the human observations.

What I find especially surprising is that almost every study produced positive results. Even when steroids were aggressively used to bring on remission, and the volunteers couldn't continue with the diet and supplements, some positive results of diet and EPA supplements were observed.

Animal studies confirmed what had been observed in human volunteers. This is important since IBD is especially frustrating to researchers because the effects of external influences, such as food and stress, are difficult, if not impossible, to control completely. The animals used in the research have no choice but to follow the diet and supplements.

The few studies in which special EPA was injected into test subjects confirmed all the other observations. This approach has been studied in Asian countries where IBD is growing rapidly, most likely due to the incredible rise in meat (especially beef) consumption.

The most rewarding observation is that many people in the clinical studies who could stick with the diet and supplement plan have remained in remission for more than two years as I write this. People who follow the plan on their own tell me the same thing. The only conclusion is that it works. If that isn't sufficient incentive to start and stick with the program I have described, I'd like to hear about the alternatives.

## Are the Results 100 Percent Effective?

If anyone ever tells you his treatment or plan works 100 percent of the time, hold on to your wallet and run. No research or treatment is 100 percent effective. In research, some studies are done incorrectly, or the design is flawed and the results are mixed at best and sometimes negative. No treatment can work all of the time because some people have been misdiagnosed and have other illnesses, or a combination of illnesses. And there are variations on these variables.

Unless the beginning hypothesis is completely correct, research on IBD diets and omega-3 oil supplements has been more successful than I would expect. I suspect this is due to the incredible difficulty in studying IBD; when a study is mounted, the design is unusually precise and the volunteers carefully diagnosed and motivated to stick to the plan. In addition, researchers have profited from mistakes made in easier similar studies of rheumatoid arthritis. I have included a listing of the research for this chapter at the end of this book for both you and your health-care provider.

If you're sufficiently curious, you can go to a medical library and start reading these papers; they will lead you to others. The experience will cement your feelings that diet can be of immense benefit to your health and will make your life more abundant.

Doctors, nurses, and other professionals often dismiss diet as an adjunct to their approach. In their own specialization they are not likely to read these papers and are usually faced with a difficult "here and now" situation. Besides, medical school curricula often don't include diet/nutrition, so physicians are unaware of it much of the time. I know because I have taught in medical schools. Show this list to your healthcare providers; better still, copy it to help them get started. They could develop some insights of their own that usually come only to clinicians who deal with these diseases. Other patients will benefit as well, and you'll be rewarded even more.

## If I Start Now, When Will I Get Results?

Read the section "Nutrition Works in Slow Motion" (page 144). You must stick with the plan through good times and bad. Eventually, as your body shifts its fat reserves and prostaglandin PGE-3 dominates, inflammation and tissue damage will begin to subside. The time between flare-ups will increase and they will be less severe. Your life will be more abundant.

## Two Sources of Research Support

Major research in the dietary control of inflammation focused first on rheumatoid arthritis, which is more widespread, a lot easier to study, and exerts a greater economic impact than IBD. It was the ideal place to start.

Inflammation in rheumatoid arthritis is visible, its impact is easily observed, and it's measured by several criteria, including use of nonsteroid anti-inflammatory drugs (NSAIDs).

The criteria used by scientists and the results are summarized as follows:

1. *Number of tender joints decreased significantly and consistently.* Joint damage (tissue damage) decreased proportionately.
2. *Morning stiffness improved.* The diet participants woke up with more flexible joints. This is a major criterion in arthritis.
3. *Time to fatigue lengthened.* People would be able to go longer without feeling tired.

4. *Grip strength improved.* This objective measure simply evaluates a person's ability to grip a device.
5. *NSAID use decreased.* In most studies, daily NSAID use decreased by 70 percent. This means that some people could stop altogether, while others used it less.
6. *Ritchie Joint Index and Global Assessment improved.* These two objective criteria are strictly clinical evaluations and are important to clinicians.
7. *Biochemical changes improved.* Prostaglandin PGE-3, the good prostaglandin, and the good leukotrienes increased as predicted by the metabolic map in Chapter Ten (page 124). The corresponding bad prostaglandin and bad leukotrienes decreased proportionately.

These findings are very important to medical scientists because they prove that the biochemical theory is correct and diet can at least control inflammation in rheumatoid arthritis. If we couple these findings with those on IBD, we can confidently conclude that diet should be a major part of IBD management.

## Nutrition Works in Slow Motion

Although the clinical studies on both arthritis and IBD were spectacular, they proved that it takes about twelve weeks for consistent results to emerge, so you have to make a serious commitment and have confidence that you will achieve the desired results. Clinical studies can never do what only you can do: follow the correct diet.

Most of the clinical studies of arthritis sufferers used either 3 or 6 grams of EPA omega-3 oil supplements daily. Indeed, the dose-response relationship was further confirmation that the supplements work. This proves that diet combined with sensible EPA and flax oil supplements can help manage IBD. What worked to reduce the inflammation of rheumatoid arthritis can work to reduce the inflammation associated with IBD.

# CHAPTER 12

# "Let Food Be Thy Medicine"

When you are diagnosed with a chronic illness like IBD, you have questions that need answers, and rightfully so. After all, what is more important than understanding the disease you are facing and learning how to keep it under control?

I've tried to anticipate some of these questions. I hope the answers will not only be helpful but also give you some guidelines on how to manage your illness.

## Can Food Help Inflammatory Bowel Disease?

As Hippocrates said in the fifth century B.C., "Let food be thy medicine." Food *can* help IBD, but it can't cure it. So be realistic, approach the disease with an open mind, and ask some questions. A questioning mind generates knowledge that will guide you to the personal responsibility associated with the disease—diet and lifestyle.

## Questions Most Often Asked About Diet Support for IBD

I've listed the most typical questions people ask me when I speak on IBD, or that I've received from people who followed the plan in my book *Eating Right for a Bad Gut*. If you have other questions, jot them down, and if they aren't answered in this book, write to my address (44 Los Arabis Circle, Lafayette, CA 94549). You will get an answer!

- Can diet cure IBD?
- What results will I experience?
- How soon will I experience results?
- How do I know it will work? Where's the proof?
- Will the plan benefit everyone?
- Can the same diet strategy work for all types of IBD?
- Can vegetarians follow the plan?
- Should I speak to my doctor first? What will my doctor say?
- Do I need to take vitamins? Will herbs help? Other supplements?
- Is the diet plan hard to follow?

## Can Diet Cure IBD?

No! As of now, nothing can cure IBD, including all modern drugs, herbs, nostrums, devices, and surgery! Diet can reduce the symptoms and flare-ups and make them less severe. Most important, it can help reduce medication by a large measure, or shift control to a milder drug. Many people will be able to stop taking daily medication and require a less potent drug if a flare-up occurs. For me, that's reason enough to follow the diet. Surgery often, but not always, stops the progression of IBD, even if the patient has to live with a pouch or colostomy, and the diet is helpful for people even after surgery.

## What Results Will I Experience?

In about two weeks or so you'll notice your symptoms are not as severe, and there is a decline in diarrhea.

In three months, you will have much more freedom from flare-ups and the pain that accompanies diarrhea. If you've been using drugs regularly or even occasionally, you'll need less.

You can't see that the damage to your intestine is slowing or has even stopped, because damage occurs gradually. You've got to have faith that you're building a better future; you're preventing further damage.

You are taking control of your health and, consequently, your destiny. Not many people take control of their lives, so taking these small steps puts you in an elite minority and should boost your self-esteem.

## How Soon Will I Experience Results?

You'll start feeling a little better within a couple of weeks. However, clinical research proves that when you stick with the program, maximum results take three months. This isn't a long time; I'll explain why.

You didn't get IBD in a day or two. Chances are you've been eating a typical diet that contains fats and oils that work against your illness. In addition, you have fat reserves that reflect the diet you've been following. You need to make some minor adjustments to your fat reserves, and that can take from six to ten weeks, depending on how aggressively you follow the plan and how heavy you are. Nutrition works in slow motion and the rewards are worth the effort.

## How Do I Know It Will Work?

You only know it won't work if you choose not to follow the plan. The old saying, "go with the winners," applies here.

In Chapter Eleven, you read about the clinical tests and

the scientific findings on which they were based. If you follow the plan you will gain some if not all of those benefits. Suppose you only gain one benefit, you don't get flare-ups as often. That alone should make it all worthwhile.

There are also psychological benefits that come from knowing you are doing your best to optimize your life.

## Does the Plan Work for Everyone?

Yes. Anyone who has IBD will experience some benefit. The sooner you start the diet, the greater the benefit will be and the less tissue damage will occur. So if you developed your IBD yesterday and you start on the diet plan today, you will gain the most benefit. If you've had IBD for ten years or more, you already have tissue damage that can't be reversed, but that shouldn't stop you from preventing further damage and flare-ups. Let your past experience be a prologue for a new life.

## Can the Same Diet Strategy Work for All Types of IBD?

Saying "all" is like saying "never." Most types of IBD sufferers will experience beneficial results from this diet plan. I'll go out on a limb and predict that people with all types of inflammatory disease will gain some relief. Maximum benefit will go to people with early-stage IBD, because they won't have to go through the suffering and tissue damage that those with more advanced IBD have experienced. Research on inflammatory disease confirms this point.

## Can Vegetarians Follow the Plan?

Vegetarians stand the best chance of success, because their dietary habits most closely match the diet plan. For example, vegetarians who use dairy products and eggs only need to

alter their fat consumption and add some supplements—
and they're 100 percent there.

## Should I Ask My Doctor First?

If you're generally healthy, you really don't need to consult your doctor; after all, this diet is good, balanced food,
and the supplements have been proven safe. There are no
foods or supplements in this plan that will interact with your
medicine or that cannot be eaten if you are allergy free. If
you do have a serious food allergy or sensitivity, you already
know what to avoid, and that applies to this plan as well as
any other. If your medication can't be used with certain
foods or food supplements, you should have been given this
information by your doctor, nurse, or pharmacist. If in
doubt, always ask your pharmacist.

## What Will My Doctor Say?

Medical doctors and foundations have a tendency to dismiss diet plans with the cliché "just eat a balanced diet."
After all, about 85 percent of illnesses will clear up with a
standard, "balanced" diet, lots of water, and rest. However,
studies from most countries have proven time and again that
less than 10 percent of "average people" eat a "balanced"
diet; in fact, the reality is more like 1 percent. The converse
of these findings is that at least 90 percent don't eat a balanced diet, and about 70 percent don't even come close.
When you have IBD, the typical "balanced diet" isn't good
enough. The dietary objective for you is to reduce some food
oils and increase others. A typical balanced diet calls for
meat and dairy products that contain those bad oils. Worse,
it allows cooking and salad oils, spreads, and shortenings
that have too much of the wrong oils. A slight shift in these
eating habits will change everything. The diet plan in this
book is balanced, but you'll still have to use supplements of
EPA, fiber, vitamins, and minerals.

If your doctor says, "Just eat a balanced diet," point out that the diet plan in this book is a special plan based on good, solid medical research. He or she should be delighted that you are doing all you can to help yourself, and you will be an "ideal patient." Your personal diet and lifestyle will have a greater impact on your health than anything else you do on a daily basis.

## Do I Need to Take Vitamins?

I use and recommend sensible supplements as described in Chapter Seven. In this case, sensible supplements support the diet and improve its effectiveness. "Sensible" starts with a multiple vitamin-mineral to ensure complete nutrition; omega-3 oil supplements (just like the ones used in many studies) to enhance the results; and a fiber supplement. Several studies indicate that most people, especially those with IBD, consume less than 50 percent of their required dietary fiber. There is some evidence suggesting that people with IBD need more fiber than the average person. Fiber is essential in the formation of solid stools and the elimination of natural wastes that are actually harmful.

## Will Herbs Help?

We are living through an herbal renaissance. People are rediscovering herbs and are using them to replace everything from vitamin pills to the family doctor. By now you know I'm a pragmatist who says, "Show me the proof." I have seen no clinical studies that indicate an herb can cure and effectively relieve the symptoms of IBD. If you know of one write to me.

Unfortunately, most herbalists are self-appointed experts who were taught by similar self-proclaimed experts. Ask to see proof of their training and then check out the school they attended. I've learned that more often than not the "expert" took a weekend or, at most, a three-week course and received a degree with a pompous title. It's your life, and if you want to trust your health to just anyone, it's your business— but be informed.

Herbs can't substitute for the diet plan in this book and they absolutely do not supply enough nutrients to replace any of the supplements I recommend.

## Is the Diet Plan Hard to Follow?

I have been advising people on diet for more than thirty-five years. I've worked with astronauts, aviators, Mt. Everest climbers, long-distance sailors, and people with chronic illnesses such as arthritis and IBD.

Not only is the plan in this book easy to follow, it will improve your health as well. All you must do is change some of your eating habits. And on life's difficulty scale that doesn't come close to living through just one flare-up. A point bears repeating: "You've got to eat, so why not select food for a more abundant life?"

# CHAPTER 13

# *Excellent Protein Sources*

## Stop Eating Red Meat

Ten to 15 percent of the calories in your new diet will come from protein. The typical person thinks of meat (beef—perhaps a nice, thick steak—pork, or veal) as the primary source of protein. Perhaps you even think of an omelet. The average person doesn't think of fish right away, even though it's the best source of protein available. A letter I received from a woman named Pat illustrates my point:

> *Dear Dr. Scala,*
> *I received your diet today and it's good news and bad news. The good news is that your scientific review convinces me it will work; the bad news is that meat is out and fish is in. Our freezer has six months of beef and lamb. My husband eats meat twice daily, but my family agreed to make the commitment with me. So I will start cooking for myself, but they will have to start later.*

To many people, protein means beef. In fact, each year the average American (as well as the average person in other Western cultures) consumes 360 pounds of red meat, 106 pounds of poultry, 250 pounds of eggs and milk, and only 23 pounds of fish. Pat's letter represents a typical response from a person who never eats fish and eats only a little poultry. If your major source of protein is meat, you must change your habit. The average American eats the equivalent of an 1100-pound steer (edible meat) every four years and eleven months. Since many people, including children, don't eat much meat at all, it means that some people are eating beef two or three times a day.

Cutting out red meat pays big dividends because your can-

---

### Eliminate
### Animal Fat

---

cer and heart disease risk will also decline. For example, epidemiologists have proven that colon cancer rates among people who eat red meat five or more times weekly is 3.5 times that of those who eat it once a month or less often. It's 1.5 times higher than those who eat red meat twice a week. Mortality rates from heart disease are similar in the same comparison. So if your family is like Pat's, everyone will gain by not eating red meat. As a person with IBD, you can gain even more.

Careful studies have shown that factors in red meat aggravate inflammation in up to 20 percent of sufferers of IBD, arthritis, multiple sclerosis, and other inflammatory diseases. This means that red meat will probably cause flare-ups, or if your IBD is chronic (always painful), red meat will make it even worse.

## Fish Is Best

It won't be as hard as you think. By following my plan, you will gradually change your eating habits so that next year you'll be consuming very little (if any) red meat. Instead you will eat lots of fish, a reasonable amount of poultry, and many more vegetables. Cutting back on milk and eggs (except for skim milk and eggs in cooking) will bring your egg and milk consumption to a reasonable level. You will obtain excellent protein from vegetables, especially beans. Your fish consumption will increase to 150 pounds or more annually! And you will find that your life is going better.

We need protein for growth, development, and body renewal, and just about all the foods we eat contain some amounts.

For example, did you know that 35 percent of the calories in mushrooms come from protein? Because there is no fat in mushrooms, the remaining 65 percent of calories come from excellent complex carbohydrates, which include some fiber.

In contrast to mushrooms, ground chuck gets 32 percent of its calories from protein and 66 percent of its calories from fat—lots of arachidonic acid—and no carbohydrate.

Compare that with a nice piece of salmon. Salmon delivers 67 percent of its calories from protein and 28 percent from fat—with up to 1.5 grams of EPA. If you eat salmon for just one meal a day and avoid meat and animal products for the other two meals, you will feel better without doing anything else. If, in addition, you take a capsule or two of EPA and use flax oil, you'll feel *very well.*

> **Fish provides the most protein
> for the least number of calories
> and the best fat distribution.**

Fish can be classified several ways. Table 13.1 lists the EPA content of some commonly consumed fish, all excellent protein sources. This dietary commitment asks you to compare them on the basis of EPA content.

### TABLE 13.1

#### EPA Content of Commonly Available Fish

| Fish (3½-ounce Serving) | EPA Content (grams)* |
| --- | --- |
| Anchovy | 0.7–1.5 |
| Striped Bass (fillet) | 0.2–0.8 |

*Includes EPA and alpha linolenic acid. The amount of EPA varies with the location of the catch, the season, and the food the fish have been eating.

| Fish (3½-ounce Serving) | EPA Content (grams)* |
|---|---|
| Cod (fillet) | 0.3 |
| Eel (fillet) | 0.4–1.0 |
| Flounder (fillet) | 0.1–0.8 |
| Herring | 1.2–2.7 |
| Halibut (fillet) | 0.3 |
| Mackerel | 0.7–2.6 |
| Sardines | 0.9–1.0 |
| Salmon (fillet) | 1.0–2.6 |
| Salmon (canned in water) | 1.1–3.2 |
| Salmon, coho | 0.2–1.0 |
| Snapper | 0.1–0.3 |
| Trout | 0.2–1.0 |
| Tuna (canned in water) | 0.4–2.6 |
| Whiting | 0.9 |
| Crab | 0.6 |
| Shrimp | 0.5 |

## Eggs Are Special

While you should really exclude eggs on this plan because of their fat content, I make an allowance because most people with IBD can eat eggs that have been soft boiled, poached, and even lightly scrambled. Eggs are your best protein purchase, and if you eat a few eggs a week, it shouldn't matter. On days you eat eggs, take an extra EPA capsule or two or add a tablespoon of flax oil.

## Use Vegetable Protein as a Meat Substitute

Thanks to modern food technology, you can purchase vegetable protein (usually from soy) in most supermarkets or mail-order it from catalogs, as either preformed burgers or a dry mix to which you add water to make "meat loaf" or burgers. I take pride in serving these soy burgers and receiving compliments from people who think they just ate a regular hamburger.

You can also purchase the soy textured as "chicken cubes" or "beef strips." Preparation is simple, and these products can be served in any dish that calls for either chicken or beef. Once I served chili made with soy "beef strips" and received compliments on its tenderness. No one realized it wasn't real beef.

The fat content of these products usually comes in at 20 to 25 percent of calories, which is the recommended level for a healthy heart. Better still, the fat content is mostly unsaturated and contains no arachidonic acid, so it's ideal.

Don't confuse soy protein products with soybean meal, which many people find distasteful and which often causes gas due to indigestible materials. Soy meal is ground soybeans, and it contains undesirable factors; for example, it contains poorly digestible starches that are digested in the lower intestine by intestinal microorganisms, which causes gas and general discomfort. Raw soy meal is not a "friendly food" for anyone, especially people with IBD; however, when it is refined and the undesirable components are removed, it provides excellent food value.

Alternatively, both beans (with rice) and egg substitutes are excellent vegetable protein sources. Remember, you only need about 60 grams of protein daily, and the chances are you are getting up to 125 grams—more than twice your need. Some experts also claim that reducing protein is healthy because it reduces the risk of kidney disease. While the scientific jury is still out on that one, the evidence keeps growing.

---

### Protein Recap

This diet plan emphasizes protein from fish. The protein plan is excellent in both quantity and quality. Sources include fish, fowl, and vegetables. Look at it this way: any food that didn't swim, fly, or grow from the ground won't be good for you. Limit sources that fly, stick to white meat, and remove fat.

# CHAPTER 14

# *Less Fat, More EPA*

About 25 percent or less of your calories should come from fat; on this diet you will minimize animal fat and reduce your polyunsaturated oil intake. Specifically, I want you to reduce arachidonic acid (animal fat) and moderate linoleic acid (found in corn oil and many cooking oils). Remember, they are the primary substances from which the antagonistic prostaglandin PGE-2 is made.

Our objective also bears repeating—to elevate dietary and metabolic eicosapentaenoic acid (EPA) to a level where it effectively competes with arachidonic acid (AA), so that your body makes more of the noninflammatory prostaglandin PGE-3 than the inflammatory PGE-2. Remember, we get EPA from fish and as food supplements; the objective of this plan is to raise EPA in your diet.

## A Few Simple Rules

- Get at least 2 grams of EPA each day in protein-rich fish and in capsules as food supplements; 5 grams is better.
- Get ALA daily by taking flax oil, preferably by adding a tablespoon to foods, or in capsules.
- Stop eating red meat and the dark meat of fowl.

- Stop using corn oil in baking. Instead, use olive oil or canola oil. Both are excellent for this diet, because olive oil is mostly a monounsaturated oil with less linoleic acid, and canola oil contains ALA and not as much linoleic acid.
- Bake, broil, barbecue, boil, poach, or microwave your food.
- Stop using egg yolks unless your serving provides a fraction of one egg. For example, a cake that uses one or two eggs and serves ten to sixteen pieces is okay. But just eat one piece!
- Stop using whole milk or any milk if it has fat in it. Skim milk and the products of skim milk are okay. Use yogurt or low-fat cottage cheese.
- Learn to use milk substitutes such as soy or rice beverage.

## A Milk Tip!

My support for skim milk has almost caused me some blackened eyes, but I've finally discovered the secret of making it palatable. Add 3 to 4 tablespoons nonfat dry milk to a quart of skim milk, which will make it thicker and creamier. This combination works well on cereal and in coffee and tea, and it has no fat!

## A Lesson in Cooking

Judge which 3½-ounce skinless chicken breast prepared two different ways is best.

A roast chicken breast provides 166 calories, of which 126 (or 76 percent) are from protein (32 grams, or half your daily needs). Only 18 percent of calories come from fat. Even though chicken has no EPA, it's okay for this plan. As a bonus, its low fat content makes it ideal for preventing heart disease.

Now purchase the same piece of chicken from a typical fast-food emporium where it is breaded and cooked in fat under pressure. The same 3½ ounces now provides 323 calories, of which 58 percent come from highly saturated, arachidonic acid–containing fat. Fifteen percent come from the breading and 27 percent from protein (22 grams).

Worse, sometimes the fat used in preparation is "lard," or simple animal fat, which is a superior source of arachidonic acid. Avoid *all* processed chicken and fish for this reason. No matter what the purveyor says about the source of the fat, the fat content is too high. More than thirty-five years in the food industry have enabled me to see their intentions more clearly now.

For example, the objective of fast-food companies is to make money by gaining market share. This means appealing to "taste" and "mouth feel," which have nothing to do with health. That is why groups such as The Center for Science in the Public Interest show that baked goods are usually laden with fat, or that soup mixes are about 20 percent salt (all cleverly hidden by manipulating ingredients lists).

The appeal to taste is a powerful factor in our diet preference. I was once invited to speak at the Executive Chefs' Association annual meeting; I spoke about how they should strive to provide more low-fat and higher-vegetarian-content meals. About six months later, one chef told me he'd been experimenting in his executive restaurant with my suggestions. In his own words, this was the result: "When I served low-fat, highly vegetarian meals, half the food went into the garbage. If instead I served fish in a rich sauce with a vegetable garnish, they licked the plate clean and left their salad. It seems that the more fat I can squeeze into a recipe, the more they like the dish."

His comments describe our tendency to enjoy the wrong tastes. However, we can retrain our taste buds to enjoy low-fat, healthy foods. It only takes a little time and a commitment to better health.

Fish and fowl are excellent sources of protein with little fat, and they are naturally balanced in sodium and potassium. We can either enhance them by broiling or barbecuing, or make them a metabolic nightmare by converting them to high-fat, high-salt foods. Food is a personal responsibility.

## EPA Supplements

Even if you decide to eat fish often, you will not get the minimum 2 grams of EPA you require daily. The best sources of EPA are oily fishes such as mackerel and anchovies, but most people don't like them. Alternatives such as salmon, tuna, and trout are often unavailable. Other fish require two or more servings to get 1 gram of EPA. Like dietary supplements of vitamins and minerals, EPA capsules are actually food in capsule form. Thanks to modern engineering, the capsules are a convenient way to make sure you get sufficient dietary EPA.

---

**Omega-3 EPA Supplements**

**3+ grams daily for adults**
**up to 3 grams daily for children**

---

If you're skeptical about taking EPA supplements, review once more the numerous clinical studies in Chapter Eleven. All used large quantities of EPA, and the results were positive. There were no negative side effects, which proves EPA is safe and effective and can provide a higher quality of life. Recognize also that in other studies related to heart disease, the subjects took 18 or more grams of EPA daily with no negative side effects. Therefore, taking up to 5 grams of EPA daily is totally safe.

## Flax Oil

Adding flax oil to your diet, even if you take EPA, will confer an additional benefit as it helps push your metabolism to produce more PGE-3. For people who are strictly vegetarian (vegan), it is completely vegetable oil. Flax oil (52 percent alpha linolenic acid or ALA) is a rich golden color, practically tasteless, and odorless. It can be purchased in liquid form in bottles, so it can easily be added to your food. Don't fry or bake with flax oil because ALA doesn't tolerate heat well. I add 1 tablespoon of flax oil to my morning bowl of oatmeal or any other cereal. Alternatively, it can be added to salad dressing or used along with vinegar, oil, and spices to make your own vinaigrette dressing. Use it on baked potatoes in place of butter and sour cream.

Flax oil is also conveniently sold in capsules. Just don't substitute flax oil capsules for EPA completely unless you're a strict vegan. For example, if you take three flax oil capsules or use a tablespoon of liquid flax oil daily, it will count as a substitute for a 1-gram EPA capsule. Because not all ALA is converted to EPA, this 3-to-1 requirement is necessary. Even if you use 3 tablespoons, or 45 grams of flax oil (the equivalent of three EPA capsules), please take one EPA capsule daily as extra insurance. I recommend this because your metabolism might not convert all the ALA in flax oil to EPA as effectively as that of a person who doesn't have IBD, so extra EPA serves as insurance. By the way, reduced heart disease and breast cancer in women are added benefits of using both EPA and flax oil.

---

**Flax Oil
3 capsules daily
(equivalent of 1 gram of EPA)**

---

## Must Vegans Use More Flax Oil?

Yes! This question often comes up when I speak on IBD. Although there are no clinical studies on flax oil similar to those presented on omega-3 in Chapter Eleven, anecdotal

reports are mounting, as you would expect. After all, research has proven that your body converts ALA from flax oil
into EPA. If you don't use EPA, I recommend 3 to 5 tablespoons of flax oil daily, since no metabolic conversion is 100
percent.

## Suppose You Don't Eat Fish

If you think you can't eat fish, don't despair. There are
many other foods you can eat. If your dietary EPA is still less
than 1 gram per day, you can simply use EPA and flax-oil supplements daily.

However, I must urge you to try fish. It's a rare individual
who can eat no fish. Learn which fish agree with you and re-
solve to like them. Experiment with different recipes, and
you'll probably discover one that suits your taste.

Of all the people who started this plan, none disliked fish
as much as Ruth and Fred. Both had emigrated from Ger-
many, and to them food meant meat, often processed meat
such as sausage. Indeed, they probably ate beef in some form
three times a day. An excerpt from Ruth's letter tells it all:

> At first I thought my IBD and your diet would bring 20 years
> of marriage to an end. I experimented with fish and vegetarian
> meals. Fred simply didn't eat them, but one day he tried some
> "salmon sausages" and admitted they were quite tasty. I no-
> ticed he's lost some weight and seems to have more energy. After
> one year on this program, he only eats meat when we go out for
> dinner.

Ruth's comment about Fred's energy is not surprising. Saturated fat (from meat) requires more oxygen to metabolize
it and reduces the body's energy production, so Fred really
did have more energy.

## Fat Recap

This diet provides adequate essential fats and emphasizes EPA from fish and supplements. Flax oil is an excellent way to achieve IBD relief, so take 2 tablespoons or its equivalent in capsules daily. A major dietary objective is to reduce total fat intake.

# CHAPTER 15

## *Complex Carbohydrates*

Sixty to 70 percent of calories in this diet come from complex carbohydrates (which is the plan everyone should follow, even if they don't have IBD). Complex carbohydrates (in contrast to sugar, a simple carbohydrate) are those that nature provides in grains, cereals, tubers, vegetables, fruits, and leafy vegetables. We also consume complex carbohydrates in processed foods such as pasta, whole-grain breads, cereals, and baked goods. It's what we do with what nature provides that counts.

Fruit sugar (usually a mixture of intensely sweet fructose and moderately sweet glucose) is an exception. Fruit sugar acts more like complex carbohydrate in your body because it's enrobed in fruit's special fiber. Fruit fiber is especially rich in pectin, which helps modulate the absorption of sugar, so be sure to eat lots of fresh fruits.

When not packaged by nature as fruits or part of other carbohydrate-rich foods (such as high-fiber cereal and high-fiber waffles and pancakes), sugar gets into our bloodstream too quickly. Excess sugar can cause mood swings, and it definitely induces your body to produce more fat. More fat means more arachidonic acid (AA), and that's not good news for your diet. Excess sugar definitely contributes to heart disease, diabetes, and other modern health problems.

Although everyone says, "Not me!", most adults consume 130 pounds of sugar each year; that's a heaping (to over-flowing) 6-ounce glass full of sugar each day. Most people use one-third of it as visible sugar (about 32 pounds a year); that's only 1.5 ounces each day—3 teaspoons or so in cof-fee or on cereal. The remaining 4.5 ounces is hidden in all the processed food we eat. For example, the 8 fluid ounces of soft drink we average each day contains almost 7 tea-spoons of sugar. Bread, desserts, and fast foods contain sugar. It is everywhere, even in salami—which is loaded with arachidonic acid and is something you should never eat again!

## Sugar Substitutes

Although there is not a smidgen of evidence to support the notion that sugar substitutes cause weight loss, they are fine if you can use them. Most people with IBD don't toler-ate low-calorie, artificially sweetened beverages well. Artifi-cial sweeteners can serve you well if you can use them, but don't delude yourself into believing you can eat more food as a reward. Rather, see them as a tool to help you reduce your inflammation. While they are considered safe, in my opinion, you should use them sparingly.

## Blood Sugar and Blood Pressure

Sugar entering the blood too quickly causes a rapid in-crease in blood sugar. The body responds to this rapid in-crease by producing insulin, a hormone that facilitates utilization of the sugar. When sugar enters the blood exces-sively fast, the insulin response is similarly excessive, and blood sugar rises quickly; then, within a short time, the blood sugar drops below normal, responding to the excess insulin. This produces a condition known as hypoglycemia, or low blood sugar.

Blood sugar influences our moods. After all, it's the only

energy source our brain has available, and when it's too low, it's a sort of primitive signal that all is not well. This leads to a number of mood changes, which range from irritability and anxiety to depression. Because 18 percent of people with inflammatory disease also suffer from depression, it's important to monitor your blood sugar level. The rule is simple: Don't use sugar in quantity or foods that contain a lot of sugar.

The omega-3 oils, specifically EPA, also have a role in depression because they help to elevate brain serotonin. Recent studies have proven that when blood levels of EPA are elevated, mild depression declines. This explains why people who followed the diet claimed they had a better outlook, and why women with premenstrual syndrome felt so much better on this diet. In both cases, the depression either cleared up or became minor. However, don't confuse the mild depression discussed here with severe clinical depression requiring close medical supervision. Severe depression is a very serious, but treatable, illness.

A lesser-known factor is the effect insulin has on your kidneys. Though this is not a problem for most people, the drugs used to treat inflammation (including IBD) increase the risk of high blood pressure as one of their side effects. So, if in addition to using medication you have elevated insulin because of eating excessive sugar, you have an above average risk of high blood pressure. Avoid sugar as much as possible as one more step toward better health.

---

## Complex Carbohydrates Recap

On this plan, carbohydrates will account for more than 60 percent of your calories. Emphasis is placed on the complex, natural carbohydrates found in fruit, vegetables, grains, and pastas. The plan helps to maintain constant blood sugar levels.

# CHAPTER 16

# *Dietary Fiber*

Our bodies produce many materials that are eliminated in urine, by way of the gallbladder, or through the intestine itself. The important thing is that the digestive system should have adequate dietary fiber available to bind up these materials and flush them from the body. Generally, this means getting 25 to 35 grams of dietary fiber each day from carbohydrate-rich foods and fiber supplements.

Fiber is also the best means of binding the loose stools of IBD and especially the bile acids. At first, many people find this incongruous with their previous knowledge because fiber is usually used to overcome constipation. Actually, fiber works both ways very effectively—it binds loose stools and will prevent constipation.

## The Selective Carrier

Fiber is like a brush with selective bristles that, in addition to moving things along, can selectively bind unwanted materials and remove them from the system. Put another way, there are five or six types of fiber, all of which have properties we require, and a varied diet provides them all. Sometimes selective supplementation helps.

Hard fiber is the "water carrier" that helps to produce regularity in most people; in excess, it can cause trouble in IBD. Some hard fiber is found in all plant food, but mostly in cereals and grains, most vegetables, beans, and tubers such as potatoes. You need to increase hard fiber to help bind up and prevent watery diarrhea.

In contrast to the hard fiber, the soluble forms of fiber, such as pectin, gums, and saponins, are the best at selective absorption and binding stools. For example, pectin helps to reduce cholesterol by binding the bile acids produced by your liver from cholesterol and removing them in your stools. Binding bile acids in IBD can eliminate much intestinal irritation. Oat bran in oatmeal does it better, and guar gum even better still. It also binds the cholesterol and fat that you get in your diet and helps to carry them through the system.

Not surprisingly, dietary fiber from fruits and vegetables also removes unhelpful by-products of metabolism, which in turn helps IBD. It appears that some materials (those produced by the body and secreted into the intestine by the gallbladder) act as antagonists and cause inflammation. The bile acids, which are strong irritants, are also bound by soluble fiber.

## Fiber from Food

An easy way to get a good start on the fiber you need is to begin each day with cereal. Many excellent cereals are available: oatmeal, bran flakes, Shredded Wheat, Wheaties, and others. Eat fruits (even canned) on cereal, on pancakes, or plain; eat more fruit along with vegetables, grains, and tubers at each meal. As your fiber intake improves, you'll have less watery and irritating stools.

High-fiber snacks are excellent all day, but drink lots of water, which increases the value of fiber. The following list contains some readily available cereals that provide sufficient dietary fiber.

*Cold Cereals*
3 to 5 grams of fiber

Cheerios
Quaker Corn Bran
Ralston Bran Chex
Kellogg's Cracklin' Oat Bran
Kellogg's Bran Flakes
Post Bran Flakes
Wheaties

*Hot Cereals*

Quaker Oats
Malt-O-Meal Hot Wheat Cereal
Ralston Cream of Wheat
Wheatena

## Fiber Supplements

In my opinion, Metamucil is the best fiber supplement. It is not likely you would take an excess. I recommend at least four servings (1 rounded tablespoon in a 6- to 8-ounce glass of water), and six servings would be better. It comes unflavored and flavored; both are fine.

Fiber supplements are usually made from psyllium hulls and are often sold as "natural vegetable laxatives" under store brand names. Mix about 1 or 2 heaping teaspoonfuls or a full tablespoon with a glass of water and drink it about thirty minutes before a meal.

## Water

In nutrition, fiber's teammate is water. Water is another essential nutrient that rarely, if ever, is taken in excess.

The relationship between water and fiber is illustrated by this example: milk contains less water than green peas. The reason you don't eat milk with a fork and drink your peas is because peas have fiber, which gives them shape and holds the water. You want fiber to do exactly that in your digestive system—give stools consistency without excess firmness.

Fiber cannot perform its cleansing action without water, but our requirement for water extends far beyond that. Indeed, next to air itself, water is the most important of all nutrients. In IBD, it is especially important for the elimination of waste materials that (in the opinion of some experts) can cause flare-ups.

## A Day with 35 Grams of Fiber

Most people, including the experts, have difficulty understanding how they can get 25 to 35 grams of fiber a day, so I've prepared the following chart. This "Day of Fiber" exceeds what most people require; for example, a 125-pound woman does fine on 25 to 30 grams daily, while her 200-pound husband needs 35 grams. Therefore, the woman could use this plan as a guide while cutting back a little here and there, but her husband should stick strictly to it.

This guide allows for many substitutions. For instance, beans and rice would be an excellent protein entrée that also provides fiber. That combination could easily substitute for a luncheon sandwich.

You cannot get too much dietary fiber. In the past thirty years, I've never observed a study in which people have gotten too much dietary fiber, and that includes those in which the volunteers took 90 grams daily.

### A Day of Fiber

| Food Item | Soluble | Insoluble | Total | Calories |
|---|---|---|---|---|
| | *Breakfast* | | | |
| Bran flakes | 1.0 | 4.0 | 5.0 | 121 |
| (with ½ cup skim milk) | | | | 93 |
| Grapefruit sections | 0.6 | 1.1 | 1.7 | 39 |
| (canned) | | | | |
| Orange juice | 1.0 | — | 1.0 | 120 |

| Food Item | Soluble | Insoluble | Total | Calories |
|---|---|---|---|---|
| **Snack** | | | | |
| Banana | 0.6 | 1.4 | 2.0 | 105 |
| **Lunch** | | | | |
| 2 slices wheat bread | 0.6 | 2.2 | 2.8 | 122 |
| Turkey slices | — | — | — | 100 |
| Spinach | 1.7 | — | 1.7 | 70 |
| Broccoli | 1.6 | 2.3 | 3.9 | 23 |
| Peach (dessert) | 0.6 | 1.0 | 1.6 | 37 |
| **Snack** | | | | |
| Apple | 0.8 | 2.0 | 2.8 | 81 |
| **Dinner** | | | | |
| Fish | — | — | — | 150 |
| Brussels sprouts | 1.6 | 2.3 | 3.9 | 30 |
| Small salad | 1.6 | 2.2 | 3.8 | 50 |
| Potato | 0.7 | 1.0 | 1.7 | 200 |
| Melon (dessert) | 0.4 | 0.6 | 1.0 | 130 |
| **Snack** | | | | |
| Pear (soft) | 0.5 | 2.0 | 2.5 | 98 |
| **Total** | **13.3** | **22.1** | **35.4** | **1,569** |

Other foods eaten during the day:

| | Calories |
|---|---|
| Spreads and condiments | 100 |
| Total daily calories | 1,669 |

This day is designed to provide enough fiber with flexibility. There's room to have other foods and accompaniments, such as wine, up to 1,900 calories for most women and 2,200 calories for men. (Women might be able to use up to 2,000 calories and men up to 2,400.) It is important to recognize that no supplemental fiber was used for purposes of illustration. If you added supplemental fiber you would gain even more control over IBD.

## Fiber Recap

Fiber can help tame the gut and contribute to general health. It is obtained from cereals, grains, fruits, and vegetables. It is also available in supplement form. There are many types of fiber and all are important for this diet to be effective; therefore, I emphasize variety.

Water is necessary as both a nutrient and a teammate of fiber. Drink lots of water.

# CHAPTER 17

# *Meal Planning*

This chapter translates the *Do's* and *Don'ts* of Chapter Six into suggestions for meals and snacks if you keep in mind the objective of no animal fat and the need for omega-3 oils. The task is easier if you visualize the times when your IBD remained in remission.

To illustrate what I mean, I'll take you through a day of how I would plan meals, recognizing that you have your own tastes and preferences.

## Breakfast: Getting Started

No matter how old you are or what you do in life, breakfast is your most important meal of the day. It will influence how you will feel all day (or night if you work nights)—so approach it with the respect it deserves.

Your objective at breakfast is to obtain complex carbohydrates, protein, and dietary fiber. Protein and fiber help maintain constant blood sugar, which is essential for an even disposition, optimistic outlook, and good intellect.

## Supplements

Morning is the ideal time to take your multiple vitamin-mineral supplement, EPA, vitamins E and C, and an appropriate amount of supplemental fiber (if you cannot eat a breakfast with 5 grams of fiber).

Calcium supplements should always be taken with meals because substances in food are essential for calcium absorption.

## Breakfast Foods

Folk wisdom teaches us to have color on our plate. So breakfast should always include some fruit, which is an easy way to accomplish this requirement. Colored fruits and vegetables provide important antioxidants. Breakfast can be fruit alone—a "fruit shake" of fruit juice blended with a banana or any combination that agrees with you. As unusual as it sounds, I've known people who blend cereals, including hot oatmeal, with apricot juice, flaxseed oil, and some fruit into a breakfast shake. Not only does it taste good, but it could almost be classified as a therapeutic food.

Remember to apply the rules we've been building: use omega-3 oil and fiber—*no* animal fat.

Fruits can make a significant contribution to your daily fiber requirement; for example, most typical fruit servings, in addition to a modest fiber cereal, supply 5 grams of dietary fiber (5 grams is about 20 percent of our daily need), and fruit fiber is excellent because it's soluble fiber that helps remove waste and irritating materials from the system. Just learn to eliminate the fiber matrix.

## Fruit Juice

A morning glass of juice provides some fiber, the mineral-electrolyte potassium, carbohydrates, and some nutrients. Always choose genuine fruit juice, not one that purports to be juice but has sugar as a major ingredient. Frozen or canned is fine and, in my opinion, orange juice is best. Read the ingredients list and ask yourself: Does it contain only the juice of real fruit? If so, excellent. Does it contain sugar or corn syrup? If so, avoid it! Salt is usually used in tomato and V-8 juice, but they are also available in "low-sodium" or "no salt added" versions.

Remember, "fresh squeezed" is usually cloudy and often tastes somewhat bland. Orange juice, apple juice, tomato juice (also low-sodium V-8), prune juice, papaya juice, grapefruit juice, and pineapple juice should contain pulp and not be clear.

## Cereal

Conduct a test. Take a piece of cereal and place it on your tongue and generate a lot of saliva. Swish it around for a few minutes. Is any significant residue left? If not, don't bother to eat it because it's probably mostly sugar or simple starch; if it leaves a definite residue, it contains what you're after in a healthful cereal—fiber. For example, corn bran, bran flakes, Cheerios, Wheaties, and Shredded Wheat leave an appropriate residue.

Next, conduct an ingredients reading test. Does the ingredients list contain sugar or corn syrup before some real cereal like corn? Is sugar or corn syrup (or both) one of the first or second ingredients? If so, don't use it!

Refer back to Chapter Sixteen to find cereals providing at least 3 grams of dietary fiber in the serving declared on the label.

I have discussed methods of preparing cereal with many people and nothing surprises me. Oatmeal with apricot nectar was suggested by a woman who cannot use milk, even though she can use soy beverage. I've tried both and they're excellent in taste and nutrition.

# Milk for Cereal, Coffee, Tea, and Drinking

I don't like skim milk because it seems watery and has a blue tinge; possibly it's my imagination, but so be it. As I stated previously, a simple way to improve skim milk is to simply add 3 or 4 tablespoons of nonfat dry milk to a quart of skim milk. There's no exact amount; simply put in enough to give it more taste and body. You can use it on cereal, in coffee or tea, and anywhere else you'd use milk. It's still fat free—no arachidonic acid—tastes good, and has a higher protein delivery. If you are sensitive to milk, it is obviously not for you.

# Eggs Versus Egg Substitutes

In Chapter Thirteen, where I discussed protein, I pointed out that eggs are an exception because of their acceptance, excellent protein, and the variety of ways they can be eaten. However, if you do a lot of baking and like to eat eggs, you should learn to use egg substitutes.

Eggs do not fit directly into this diet, but egg substitutes are readily available; however, beware—some contain more fat than eggs! Just remember to read the nutritional label.

My preferences are Egg Beaters or Scramblers. Both permit you to have scrambled eggs and omelets, which should include well-cooked vegetables, especially zucchini, mushrooms, and spinach, and wheat germ. I have served mushroom and spinach omelets made from Egg Beaters to nutritionists and not one could tell that I didn't use eggs!

The addition of 1 ounce of skim-milk mozzarella cheese will add texture and body to the omelet. Although it is better to eat strictly vegetarian omelets without cheese, indulging once in a while is fine. Be sure that the vegetables have been precooked to softness before making the omelet.

## Pancakes, Waffles, and French Toast

Pancakes and waffles can be made with skim milk, Egg Beaters for eggs, and canola oil for shortening. The mix used should emphasize wheat or buckwheat flour as much as possible. Aunt Jemima mixes are my favorites, and they work fine with Egg Beaters.

Once the batter is prepared, spoon it onto the griddle and add canned sliced fruit on top—I enjoy canned sliced peaches, but peeled apples and bananas work equally well. Of course, you can also use fruit with waffles if you blend it in a food processor before adding it to the batter.

French toast made with slightly dry sourdough bread (crust removed) that is soaked overnight in dilute Egg Beaters batter using skim milk and a tablespoon of frozen orange juice concentrate is excellent. Some people use a little orange liqueur and almond extract, which adds a nice flavor and tastes delicious. The alcohol evaporates during cooking, so it is not a problem.

Toppings for pancakes, waffles, and French toast should not include butter. The American classic, maple syrup, is excellent, but so is blueberry or boysenberry syrup, or some other natural syrup.

## Morning and Afternoon Breaks

Tea is a good beverage, and juice is even better. More important is the "break snack." If you take a snack, at least choose one that provides fiber and complex carbohydrates. If that sounds like peeled fruit, it is! Don't eat doughnuts or sweet rolls because they elevate blood sugar only to let you down later. They are also rich in omega-6 oils. If you choose a muffin, make it a bran or carrot muffin. Remember, 18 percent of IBD patients also suffer from anxiety and depression—don't aggravate this tendency with bad snacking habits. This is one more reason to keep caffeine in check by drinking tea, not coffee. Excess caffeine stimulates the central nervous system but also speeds fatigue, and fatigue feeds depression.

# Lunch

Lunch is often the main meal of the day, but whatever the circumstances, it should accomplish several objectives:

1. EPA can be obtained from fish or as a supplement. Fish can be eaten as a tuna salad or sandwich, a nicely poached salmon, a grilled swordfish steak, or even smoked trout. The only variables are lifestyle and economics. With a little imagination, fish can be eaten almost every day at lunch. With a little enthusiasm, some imagination, and willpower, you can take the bad fat out of lunch and put the good EPA in.
2. Protein is always one major lunchtime objective; though not stated as such, it is often the luncheon entrée feature in restaurants. Protein can be fish, a fish garnish on pasta, shredded chicken over rice in a Chinese dish (with no MSG), and so on. There is no end to the variety. The rules of preparation must be carefully followed.
3. Complex carbohydrate is important, especially the complex carbohydrate in rice, beans, vegetables, fruits, grains, cereals (such as well-cooked wheat), and breads. This carbohydrate will provide the energy to carry you for the rest of the day and into the evening. Potatoes (skin removed) and rice are excellent choices since neither one causes intestinal problems.
4. Dietary fiber, which is obtained from complex carbohydrate—especially in fruits and vegetables—is also important.
5. Just before lunch is an excellent time to take a fiber supplement; with lunch, take one-third of your EPA supplements. You should also take one-third of your calcium supplements.
6. Green leafy vegetables, such as spinach (cooked soft), should be part of every lunch whenever possible. Tomatoes are excellent if you are careful to have them peeled, cooked, and pureed into a sauce.

## Power Lunches in a Blender

Soy protein isolates (protein that has been removed from the soy flour and contains no soy oil and very little carbohydrate) can be purchased as a protein mix that usually has a nutritional delivery similar to the following nutritional table:

**Nutrition Facts**

Serving Size 4 Rounded Tablespoons (28.4g—approximately 1 heaping scoop)

Servings Per container 17

| Amount Per Serving | Powder | Powder with 1 Cup Skim Milk |
|---|---|---|
| **Calories** | 100 | 200 |
| **Calories** from Fat* | 0 | 8 |

| % Daily Value** | | |
|---|---|---|
| **Total Fat** 0g* | 0% | 2% |
| Saturated Fat 0g | 0% | 2% |
| **Cholesterol** 0mg | 0% | 2% |
| **Sodium** 200mg | 8% | 14% |
| **Potassium** 200 mg | 6% | 20% |
| **Total Carbohydrate** 8g | 3% | 7% |
| Dietary Fiber 0g | 0% | 0% |
| Sugars 0g | | |
| **Protein** 16g | 30% | 50% |

Following will be a list of vitamins and minerals that provide from 20% to 130% of the RDI.

*Amount in Powder
**Percent Daily Values are based on a 2,000 calorie diet. Your daily values may be higher or lower depending on your calorie needs.

|  | Calories | 2,000 | 2,500 |
|---|---|---|---|
| Total Fat | Less than | 65g | 80g |
| Sat Fat | Less than | 20g | 25g |
| Cholesterol | Less than | 300mg | 300mg |
| Sodium | Less than | 2,400mg | 2,400mg |
| Total Carbohydrate |  | 300g | 375g |
| Dietary Fiber |  | 25g | 30g |
| Calories per gram: |  |  |  |
| Fat 9 | •    Carbohydrate 4 | •    Protein 4 |  |

Blend this powder with a cup of orange juice or other non-sugared fruit juice and some well-ripened banana, canned sliced peaches, orange sections, or even sliced mango. You can also mix it with soy beverage for a creamier texture and more protein. A lunch like this delivers excellent vegetable protein, very little fat, and a reasonable amount of fiber. Add a tablespoon of flax oil and you will increase your omega-3 oils.

An advantage is derived from the vegetable protein, which supplies a generous portion of nonessential amino acids that your body will use for energy later. These nonessential amino acids provide stamina, the long-term energy that keeps you going when others are tired.

## Dinner

Traditionally dinner is the family gathering time, even in today's fast-paced world in which most, if not all, people eat at least one or two meals away from home. It is a chance to talk over the day's activities, congratulate one another, identify solutions to problems that emerged, and share general fellowship. It is also a chance to improve your health while enjoying a good meal and a good time to take some supplements.

The diet plan discussed here for IBD is low in the fat that

increases heart disease and cancer, and rich in those food components, including the good fat, that prevent heart disease, reduce the risk of cancer, and increase and enhance the quality of your life. The food habits this plan instills in children will contribute to a longer, healthier life for them.

It is imperative that dinner be appealing and provide foods rich in EPA. Thus the protein source chosen for the entrée is very important. While being healthy, it should also taste good and be as elaborate as you wish to make it. Trout stuffed with mushrooms, bread, onions, and scallions sautéed in olive oil laced with garlic is one of my favorites. But just as good is a piece of broiled frozen swordfish, or on a hot day, a tuna salad. If it's not fish, it can be as varied as pheasant, skinned breast of chicken or turkey, veal, and so on. Don't forget that once a month a red meat can be an entrée.

Dinner should always include a good source of complex carbohydrate, such as rice, potato, squash, carrots, wheat, corn, barley, or millet. Pasta is always excellent and can be the major part of the meal, providing both protein and carbohydrate when served with a light tomato sauce including chicken, fish, or some other high-protein source.

Green vegetables, such as string beans, asparagus, broccoli, spinach, and turnip greens, can be boiled, steamed, or baked until soft. Soft cooked spinach with a little olive oil added before serving can be a dinner standby. For a variation, try soft cooked cabbage—there are almost endless varieties—which retains its excellent protective phytochemicals.

No dinner is complete without dessert—a tradition in many cultures. It has always been the children's reward associated with cleaning their plate, and by the time we're adults, it's habit—something we expect. Nutritionally it often provides calcium as cheese, or a fermented milk product.

Many desserts that can be made or purchased are completely acceptable on this plan. Fruit is the most natural and obviously excellent, but soft pies, such as pumpkin, sweet potato, and lemon, are fine and you may enjoy even peach and apple pies. Cream pies and most puddings are not a good choice because they contain sources of arachidonic acid. Cakes are good dessert choices when they are made with canola oil.

## Dining Out

Dining out affords an opportunity to try new things, to give the people around us an opportunity to eat something different. All you have to do is follow the *Do's* and *Don'ts* in Chapter Six.

Assert yourself by telling your waiter that you are on a special diet, and if you see something on the menu that looks good, ask questions. For example, in an Italian restaurant ask if they have a nonmeat sauce, and can the chef put it through a blender? Can sole meunière be prepared in olive oil, not butter? The possibilities become endless if you're willing to ask questions and assert your role—that of a customer!

Most chefs can prepare excellent vegetarian meals, and frozen fish is available everywhere. If you think fresh fish is always used in fine restaurants, let me describe an experience I had while at a meeting of the Nutrition Foundation in Naples, Florida.

We were eating at an expensive restaurant that emphasized seafood. Since it was in Florida, and they had scrod (a cold-water fish) as the day's special, I asked the waitress, "How do you get fresh scrod in Naples, Florida?"

Her reply startled everyone who had been extolling the excellent fresh fish: "None of our fish is fresh; it's all selected as fresh, frozen at sea."

Since then I've spoken to many people who fish for a hobby and freeze what they catch, because in their words "it gives the fish a better texture."

Beyond the entrée, the rest is easy because it's vegetables, rice, fruits, salad, and all things that are on the *Do* list. It is the preparation that's most important. Most restaurants will be glad to have the chef boil some vegetables; for dessert, a poached pear is seldom a problem.

Breakfast can be oatmeal, and if it's microwaved (ask), simply have them cook it a little longer. Avoid the raisins and toppings that often come as a garnish.

Many restaurants make "Egg Beaters" omelets or even an "egg white" omelet. However, a couple of eggs each month won't hurt, especially if you're taking EPA and using flax oil. Meanwhile, more and more restaurants are leaning toward dishes recommended by the American Heart Association, and these dishes, marked on the menu with a healthy heart symbol, are usually low in animal fat, generous in complex carbohydrate, and good sources of protein. Still others are offering "health" menus that emphasize fish, vegetables, and lighter, yet filling, dishes.

Call before you venture out to a restaurant and ask what's available. I think you'll be surprised to hear how willing many chefs are to facilitate your request.

Make notes now in your diary—what you eat, what you've eliminated, any problems or flare-ups, how you feel, how often you need medication, and so on. After a few months into your new diet plan, see how far you've come.

# PART III

# Applied Nutrition and Lifestyle for IBD

Nutrition information abounds in the news media. In fact, what you hear today will be contradicted tomorrow, and a third version will appear next week. It is a daunting task for anyone, let alone a person with IBD, because certain nutrition basics are essential to health and longevity. More important, young people with IBD are especially vulnerable to nutritional shortfalls.

This section is not a comprehensive primer on nutrition. My objective here is to present certain basic concepts you must understand if you want to thrive as opposed to simply survive. Finally, if you are a parent whose child has IBD, these basics are even more meaningful if your child is to achieve his or her full potential.

The information I have provided is scientifically sound, will stand the test of time, and is basic to good health. Please take it seriously. You are welcome to write to me if you have any questions, and you can count on me to respond.

# CHAPTER 18

# *Basic Calorie Nutrition*

Experience has taught me that people who have IBD are often on the lean side. The "leanness" relates to how severe their problems are and how frequently they flare up. In addition, when I'm speaking to groups, I can usually spot individuals with serious IBD as the men are often shorter than average, and sometimes both the men and women look a little pallid.

On the other hand, people whose IBD is not as serious and have only occasional flare-ups look more like average people. Indeed, I have even met some who should diet to lose weight.

Both are examples of how this disease works. The thin, sometimes short person could simply be showing the result of insufficient calories with the correct balance among fat, protein and carbohydrates. In a sense, it is a symptom of malnutrition: they have always "gotten by," but haven't achieved their full potential.

In contrast, the overweight IBD patient often eats the wrong food. As one physician with IBD once said, "We're all junk food junkies." What he meant was that IBD patients tend to eat highly processed foods that have lots of calories, little fiber, the wrong kind of fat, and mediocre to poor nutrition.

My objective in this chapter is for you to gain a basic understanding of how many calories you need daily and how to spread them over the three major nutrients: protein, fat, and carbohydrate. If you eat correctly, you will optimize your health. First, let's start with the calorie itself.

## What Is a Calorie?

A Calorie is the amount of energy needed to raise 1 gram of water (20 percent of a teaspoon) 1 degree on the centigrade scale. So as you might guess, a Calorie is a small amount of energy. That's why we use units of 1,000 Calories or the kilocalorie in nutrition (we all learned the 1,000 formula in school). Kilo means one thousand. It was cumbersome saying kilocalorie all the time, so it was shortened to *Calorie* instead. (It doesn't make any difference in our discussion, but when you look up food values and see *KC* or *kilocalories,* you'll know what it all means.) A Calorie measures the energy-producing value of food when oxidized in the body.

Nutritionists use a capital *C* when writing Calorie (in our discussion we will use the lowercase—calorie).

## The Optimum Diet

If you could take an average day's food, blend it together, and remove the water, you'd be left with about 1 pound— 454 grams—of dry material. Several grams would be the macrominerals—calcium, phosphorus, potassium, sodium, and magnesium. One more gram would be taken up by the vitamins and the trace minerals. That leaves 450 grams, almost the entire pound, for protein, fat, carbohydrate, and fiber. It's especially important to get these four macronutrients in the correct proportions.

An optimum proportion provides 10 to 15 percent of its calories from protein, 30 percent or fewer of its calories from fat, and the remaining 50 to 60 percent of calories as carbohydrate. In addition, you should get from 25 to 40 grams of fiber each day depending on your size.

To get these nutrients into more realistic units, let's do some basic calculations.

## Dietary Calorie Calculations

Protein and carbohydrate each provide 4 calories per gram; fat provides 9 calories per gram. So, if we work out the optimum diet for a person who needs 2,000 calories daily, we'll come up with the following:

**Protein** [Take 12% of calories (c) as average]
$12\% \times 2,000 = 240$ c $\div$ 4 c/gram          =    60g
**Fat**
$30\% \times 2,000 = 600$ c $\div$ 9 c/gram          =    67g
**Carbohydrate**
$58\% \times 2,000 = 1,160$ c $\div$ 4 c/gram      = 290g

|  |  |
|---|---|
| Total by weight | 417g |
| Fiber | 30g |
| Total with fiber | 447g |
| Total for vitamins and minerals | *about* 5g |
| GRAND TOTAL | 452g |

One pound is 454 grams. Thus, the person burning 2,000 calories daily eats about a pound of food. Since most food is about 75 percent water, the wet weight will be more than 1,800 grams; that's about 4 pounds! It seems like a lot.

Let's look at the food consumed by three different 30-year-old people: an active woman of about 120 pounds, an active person weighing about 155 pounds, and a person, probably a man, weighing about 200 pounds. The calorie distribution is shown in Table 18.1:

## TABLE 18.1

### Calorie Distribution for Three People

|  | 120 lb | 150 lb | 200 lb |
|---|---|---|---|
| Calories | 2,000 | 2,700 | 3,500 |
| Protein (12% cal) | 60 g | 81 g | 105 g |
| Fat | 67 g | 90 g | 117 g |
| Carbohydrate | 290 g | 92 g | 508 g |
| Fiber | 30 g | 35 g | 40 g |
| Nutrients | 5 g | 5 g | 5 g |
|  |  |  |  |
| Grand total dry weight | 452 g | 603 g | 775 g |
| Approximate wet weight | 1,808 g | 2,412 g | 3,100 g |
| In pounds | 4 lb | 5.3 lb | 6.8 lb |

## Variation

While you're looking over Table 18.1, think about several things. Larger people eat more food because they need more calories. If food provides all the necessary nutrients at 1,200 calories, it will provide the same at 2,000 calories. Two people who weigh the same aren't always the same height and don't always have the same shape. Some seem to be full of energy and always active, whereas others seem somewhat lethargic, inactive, and pensive. Do they all need the same calories and nutrients? No—there's a lot of variation in our requirements.

## What Influences Calorie Variation?

You already know intuitively that size, shape, activity, stress, climate, and your state of health influence your nutritional needs. The optimum diet for one person wouldn't necessarily be exactly the same for another person. For example, if you're an active 120-pound woman, you might require more than 2,000 calories daily. In contrast, if you weigh 120 pounds but sit a lot and don't exercise, you might do just fine on 1,600 calories. If you were to eat 2,000 calories you'd slowly put on weight. Why? Because our body stores extra calories as fat; every extra 3,500 calories gets stored as 1 pound of fat. Let's explore briefly where the calories go.

## Where Do Calories Go?

Everything we do burns calories. Eating and digesting food takes energy. While you're sleeping you burn about 80 calories per hour. If you run ten miles in an hour, you burn about 900 calories. Let's get back to the sleeping calories: even while you sleep your body requires energy, because it never stops running; that's basal metabolism.

## Basal Metabolism

The energy you burn to keep your system going is called basal metabolism, because it's the basic process that keeps your body systems working. For example, your normal temperature is 98.6°F; your heart beats; your kidneys continually clean wastes from your blood (about 50 gallons of blood are processed per day); your mind is always working; you breathe; and so on. These processes take place as long as you're alive and account for most of the energy you use. Basal metabolism, like money, never sleeps!

Basal metabolism varies for each of us. It's influenced by age, sex, state of health, body surface area, and stress. I'll explore each of these factors briefly to show you how they change basal metabolism; but first, how much energy does it account for?

A 120-pound woman 5 feet tall has a basal metabolic rate, called BMR, of 1,260 calories; if she's 5 feet 7 inches and 120 pounds, it's 1,360 calories. On average, the BMR for a 120-pound woman is 1,300 calories. The BMR for men the same size would be 1,350 and 1,450, respectively; 1,400 calories on average. Return to the example in Table 18.1 of the 120-pound woman who consumes 2,000 calories per day. Her

BMR, at 1,300 calories, accounts for 65 percent of her total daily energy expenditure! BMR is where most of her energy goes. Since most of everyone's energy is spent on simply staying alive, let's see what increases or decreases BMR.

From my example, it's clear that a long, thin person (5'7") burns more energy than a short (5'0") person of the same weight. One of the reasons for this energy expenditure is body shape; the shorter and rounder you are, the lower your BMR; conversely, the taller and thinner you are, the higher your BMR. This difference relates to surface area. Your body radiates heat, so the more surface you have, the more energy is lost to the atmosphere. Hence, a short, round person burns less energy than a tall, skinny person who weighs the same. Though only 1 calorie per pound doesn't sound like much, it can make a big difference over the twenty-four hours in a day.

Metabolic rate declines with age by about 2 percent per year. For instance, a person 50 years old requires about 35 percent fewer calories than a 30-year-old person. Thus, if we keep eating at age 50 as we did at age 30, we'll be getting many more calories than we need. That's why many people who insist they don't eat a lot still get fat as they get older. As we age, our perception of portion size should change, because we don't need as much food.

Metabolic rate also varies with your state of health. For example, if you are sick and running a fever, you'll require more calories to maintain a higher body temperature. But an illness doesn't have to cause a fever to increase the metabolic rate, because the body is under stress and must work to eliminate the illness or overcome its effects. Stress increases BMR even if you're not sick. In other words, if you're sick, or if you've got a chronic illness such as IBD, you'll generally use more basal metabolic calories. As a general rule, the folks I've met who have IBD aren't overweight; in fact, they usually appear slightly thinner than average. Remember, 50 percent of Americans are overweight, so as a group, people with IBD could be somewhat healthier since excess weight shortens life.

Unlike being underweight, being overweight is simple to deal with. Extra weight can be managed by controlling calories. I know there are people who claim their excess weight is the result of glands gone awry and other problems. However, if you eat fewer calories than you burn, you will lose weight. I know this goes against some notions and even what sympathetic health professionals say, but it is the absolute truth.

## Where Do the Other Calories Go?

People generally don't burn nearly as many calories as they think. For example, most people about 5 feet 4 inches tall burn about 500 calories over the BMR in a twenty-four-hour period. Add another 200 calories for digesting their food, and they've got their 2,000 calories per day. Table 18.2 lists some typical physical activities that account for some of the 500 calories average people burn.

### TABLE 18.2

### Calorie Costs
### (150-Pound Person)

| Activity | Calories per Hour |
| --- | --- |
| Resting | 80 |
| Driving | 120 |
| Housework | 180 |
| Walking 2.5 mph | 210 |
| Gardening | 220 |
| Tennis (singles) | 600 |
| Cycling 13 mph | 660 |
| Running 10 mph | 900 |

Table 18.2 shows the calories burned for a 150-pound person. A 120-pound person would burn about 20 percent less and a 180-pound person would burn 20 percent more for the same activities. If you're realistic, you'll see that in a ten-hour period, you're unlikely to burn more than 500 extra calories. For example, few women do housework nonstop; similarly, most joggers don't keep it up for more than about 20 minutes.

## Alcohol

Alcohol is between carbohydrate and fat in its calorie content. It provides 7 calories per gram. A 6-ounce glass of wine—that's 12 percent alcohol—provides 125 calories; 1.5 ounces of whiskey contain 100 calories. Both also provide a few calories from the sugar they contain.

An adult can consume up to 1½ percent of his or her daily calories from alcohol without any adverse effects. At 2,000 calories a day, that's about one glass of wine, one mixed drink, or a bottle of beer. Above that level, alcohol begins to have adverse effects.

Adverse effects of alcohol derive from its toxic nature. Since alcohol is a toxic material, the body marshals all its resources to metabolize it. If there's an excess, the body can't handle it rapidly enough and the alcohol gets to the brain, where it causes impaired function. Keep alcohol to less than 2 percent of calories, and you'll have no problem—that's one glass of wine, mixed drinks, or beer daily.

## Put All These Calories Together

In Table 18.3 I have summarized a twenty-four-hour calorie distribution for four people with IBD—a 120-pound woman, a 150-pound man and woman, and a 180-pound man—so that you can see the difference in daily calorie needs.

By studying Table 18.3 and/or using some calculations,

you can determine where you fit in. For example, for a woman weighing 135, the closest weight on Table 18.3 is 120; take the ratio of 135/120 (135 divided by 120) which equals 1.13—then multiply 1.13 times 2,087 (calories for a 120-pound woman) and you will get 2,358 calories for a 135-pound woman. Similarly, for a man weighing 200, the number of calories would be 200/180 times 2903 (or 1.11 times 2903), which is 3,222 calories. Your values will be close enough for planning. You'll see that the majority of your calories go to basic body functions. It's important to remember that if you want to increase your calorie expenditures, you've got to add an extra physical activity to your day.

I'll use myself as an example. I exercise on either a rowing machine (Nordic Row) or a simulated cross-country ski machine (Nordic Track) for 25 minutes five times weekly. Each session burns about 300 calories. That is a typical example of healthy exercise.

## TABLE 18.3

### Caloric Requirements of IBD Patients

### (Weight in Pounds)

| Weight | 120 | 150 | 150 | 180 |
|---|---|---|---|---|
| Height | 5'4" | 5'6" | 5'6" | 6' |
|  | Woman | Woman | Man | Man |
| BMR | 1,327 | 1,478 | 1,588 | 1,836 |
| Daily activity | 500 | 600 | 650 | 700 |
| Assimilation | 160 | 200 | 200 | 220 |
| For IBD illness 8% | 100 | 118 | 127 | 147 |
| Total: | 2,087 | 2,396 | 2,565 | 2,903 |

## How Accurate Is All This?

We live in a constantly changing environment. When it's cold more calories are burned to keep your body temperature at 98.6°F; when it's hot, you produce sweat to cool it down. So when I say that someone burns 2,000 calories a day, it's an average. That means some days you'll burn 1,800, other days 2,200. Therefore, you shouldn't be concerned about a variance of 100 or 200 calories on any single day. It's what we do on average that counts. We know if we're getting it right by whether we gain or lose weight.

## Why We Gain and Lose Weight

If we burn more calories on average than we eat as food, we lose weight. In contrast, if we consume more calories on average than we burn, we gain weight. Notice that I said *on average*. That's because it doesn't happen in one day; it takes many days, even months or years for the extra calories to accumulate.

Each extra pound of fat accounts for about 3,500 calories. So if you consume, on average, an extra 35 calories per day, you'd hardly notice it because it would take at least three or more months to gain an extra pound, and your scale is not that accurate. What you might notice is that something fits a little tightly.

In contrast, suppose you're eating the same foods every day and losing weight. The same number of calories are involved, but now it's a deficit, not an excess. The weight loss could mean that your basal metabolism has increased. Basal metabolism usually increases because of emotional stress or illness. If you've got IBD, the weight loss could relate to a period of diarrhea or a flare-up. The reason could be a decline in your body's ability to absorb nutrients, especially fat. When unknown or unwanted weight loss occurs, it's important to identify the cause. If you notice that you've lost a few pounds, if your clothes are looser, think about what has happened. You've created a calorie deficit of 3,500 calories for each pound—that's if you were carrying some extra body fat. But suppose you're a person without extra fat and you experience an unknown weight loss. The mathematics gets more confusing, but I'll explain it.

## Lean Body Mass

We call muscle and bones, including our carbohydrate reserves, lean body mass. This mass of protein and carbohydrate also holds about three times its weight in water. So losing a pound of protein or carbohydrate reserves drops about 4 pounds; three of water and one of protein or carbohydrate. Protein and carbohydrate each require 4 calories per gram. So once your body fat reserves are low, you can drop a pound of carbohydrate, with a deficit of only 1,800 calories, and lose 4 pounds! That's because for each pound of carbohydrate, there's about 3 pounds of water.

Once you've used your carbohydrate reserves, you start to lose protein—or muscle mass. Losing protein is dangerous and can seriously impair your health. That is why unwanted weight loss should not be taken lightly.

This type of weight loss is bad because you're losing very important body tissues and reserves that your body needs to function. Just remember that whenever unplanned weight loss occurs, discuss it with your doctor. It's important.

## Special Concerns for IBD

Three conditions of IBD make weight maintenance especially important: absorption due to intestinal inflammation, loss of calorie nutrients due to diarrhea, and poor eating habits that result from avoiding problem foods and selecting highly processed foods, or from a serious flare-up. Any one of these conditions can cause unwanted weight loss; all three together can spell disaster if something isn't done.

IBD patients often have chronic minor, if not serious, inflammation of the intestine and that causes a decrease in absorption. Indeed, people who have a "pouch" or "colostomy" sometimes notice that their food comes out exactly as it went in. Obviously the calorie nutrients, let alone other nutrients, haven't been absorbed. So, even if there is no flare-up thanks to the pouch, there is still a nutritional challenge.

Another challenge associated with IBD is diarrhea. Soft,

watery stools often contain excessive bile acids. Excessive bile acids cause malabsorption of fat. It's a serious concern because during diarrhea, you need the calories; in fact, you need more calories.

Finally, the flare-up creates a situation that causes people to stop eating. A list of supplemental food products to help you avoid malnutrition appears in Chapter Eight. Your doctor may resort to tube feeding and, as a last resort, total parenteral nutrition (TPN).

Nature provides an opportunity to overcome the calorie challenge by the use of extra calories. Fat is nature's most concentrated source of calories. Just select fats that won't compromise your health.

# CHAPTER 19

# *Protein*

In the nineteenth century, scientists identified an essential nitrogen-containing substance in food that they called *protein,* from the Greek word *proteios,* meaning "of prime importance." All animals, from mice to people, require protein. Now we know that what we really need are amino acids, which are the building blocks of protein.

## Essential Versus Nonessential Amino Acids

About twenty-two amino acids that are found throughout nature are used to make the protein of body tissues, make hormones, transport fat, and make other proteins, such as the enzymes that digest food. Indeed, any body tissue, body function, or body process involves proteins. So it follows that the basic building blocks, the amino acids, are critical.

Think of the amino acids as twenty-two different beads that can be linked together in any arrangement, and this string of amino acid beads is a protein. Since there are twenty-two amino acids and no limit to how they can be arranged in protein, it follows that there's no limit to the types of protein that can exist.

Of the twenty-two amino acids, your body can make all but eight, which we appropriately call *essential* amino acids.

These eight *essential* amino acids determine the quality of a protein. If you didn't get enough of one of the *essential* amino acids, your body wouldn't be able to make all the protein it needs; this would limit how well you'd live and possibly cause death. Nonessential amino acids are also important, and are similarly used for making protein. The nitrogen they provide is also used in many other body chemicals and tissues, including your genetic material. Normally you get a generous supply of the nonessential amino acids from food, so your body doesn't use energy to make them. They're very important in your diet, helping you thrive and not just survive. In fact, some of them are also used for energy.

But in fact, we don't eat amino acids, we eat protein. So protein that contains a good balance of the *essential* and nonessential amino acids is of better quality than protein that doesn't contain this balance. We'll come back to this point shortly, but first consider the obvious question: Why not just eat amino acids?

## Why Not Eat Amino Acids?

Actually, you *do* eat amino acids. Protein is digested in your stomach and reduced to its amino acids in the small intestine, so that they can be absorbed from the small intestine into the blood. They are then used to make body proteins and other materials, and are even used for energy. Thus it's only desirable to bypass the digestive process under special conditions where a physician and dietitian are usually involved.

Sometimes in IBD when the digestive system has flared up and must rest, or is not functioning, a doctor will prescribe an *elemental diet.* These diets, usually specially prepared under very rigorous conditions, provide all the components of food in their elemental form. These components include amino acids, some peptides, and special fats and carbohydrate as their basic elements. These medicinal foods allow the body to be nourished without digestion. In routine cases the diets are taken by mouth; in more advanced cases they are tubed directly into the stomach as enteral nutrition (EN); and in the most sophisticated diet form, total parenteral nutrition (TPN), the elements are pumped directly into the blood. TPN solutions contain the amino acids along with all the other nutrients, and while they require specialized medical supervision at first, once established, they can be personally administered at home.

Satisfying your protein requirement by purchasing pills or powders of amino acids is very costly and it requires a complex juggling of the amounts of one amino acid versus another. In fact, to do it correctly would require the supervision and practical experience of a specialized registered dietitian.

So, you ask, "What about the amino acids we see for sale in health food stores, drugstores, and some supermarkets?" Those amino acids are generally sold for *perceived* rather than *real* needs. They are usually sold to bodybuilders on the notion that they will supply an extra protein-building capacity. Some evidence suggests that bodybuilders can get *slightly* better results from their weight lifting if they use lots of protein under just the right conditions. However, the notion of taking pills of amino acids for that purpose totally lacks substance.

## Protein Quality

Protein quality is determined by the amount of each essential amino acid it contains. The old saying "a chain is as strong as its weakest link" is a good description. The quality of a protein can't be any better than the limiting amount of any one of the essential amino acids. Actually, some proteins are better than others when the amounts of each of the essential amino acids are precisely relative to the others. We say this amino acid distribution is excellent, and animal proteins are generally of the highest quality. In fact, a system of determining protein quality has been established with cow's milk protein, casein, as its standard, and a "protein standard" is kept at the National Bureau of Standards for this purpose.

The standard measure for protein quality is determined by how well young newly weaned laboratory rats grow. Because they are already growing rapidly, the protein quality is immediately obvious if the rats' growth rates improve or falter. With rapid growth as a criterion, protein sources can be conveniently graded.

If a protein is as good or better than casein, we set the adult requirement at 45 grams daily; if it's less than casein, we set the requirement at 65 grams. In everyday terms that means if you weigh about 150 pounds, you should get at least 45 grams of good-quality protein daily. Alternatively, the same 150-pound person should get 65 grams, or about 2½ ounces, if the protein quality is less than that of casein.

## Protein as Food

The proteins provided by eggs, meat, fish, fowl, and dairy products are of sufficiently good quality, so you could get along on any one of them as your only protein source even if your diet was terribly boring. However, once you look past animal (include fish) protein sources to vegetable sources, meeting your protein need requires a little more care.

Many vegetable foods provide good protein, but fall short in one or more of the essential amino acids. Since these proteins need to be complemented with other protein, we call them complementary protein foods. They include grains, nuts, beans, and peas—the legumes. None of them can serve as the sole source of protein, because you'll fall short of one or more essential amino acids. So, you have to know how to mix them to get enough protein. Because vegetable proteins are seldom adequate by themselves and must be complemented, variety is important for vegetarians. If you mix beans with rice, the rice makes up the shortcoming of the beans and vice versa. The protein mixture is then complete. Alternatively, eat milk with cereal, or yogurt with beans; the extra essential amino acids in the dairy products will complement the shortfall in the grains or beans. Similarly, if you are not vegetarian, eggs, meat, fish, and fowl complete these complementary proteins. It usually takes just a little animal protein to complement vegetable protein; for example, a meal of rice with a small amount of chicken or eggs is an excellent protein source.

Protein in each meal doesn't need to be nutritionally complete. It's the average that counts. Let's say you have cereal for breakfast, some fish or fowl at lunch, and pasta at dinner. You'll get protein from the cereal, grain (pasta), and fish. But most important, the fish at lunch will provide enough extra essential amino acids to make up for the shortfall in the pasta and cereal. If you have milk or soy beverage with the cereal, you've gained added nutritional insurance. In this case, we could call it protein insurance.

Most vegetables and fruits are insignificant sources of protein, but we recognize that we need them for other equally important purposes, and the small amount of protein they do provide contributes to the daily total.

## Meat as Condiment

This brief review of protein teaches that the best-quality protein comes from animal foods and that vegetable protein is often incomplete. Most of humanity thrives as virtual vegetarians because they use fish, fowl, eggs, dairy, and meat products as *condiments* with their legumes, rice, and other vegetarian foods. The essential amino acids in small amounts of animal protein can be enough. Think of this the next time you eat Chinese, Thai, or even haute French foods.

## Protein as Energy

Through a complex series of interactions, excess non-essential amino acids are converted to carbohydrate. After a protein-rich meal, people sometimes feel satisfied for many hours or most of a day. This results from the extra amino acids being converted to carbohydrate and getting used for energy. Eating excess protein is wasteful, however, because it gets used for energy rather than building tissue; carbohydrate and fat are the preferred sources of energy.

Excess protein means your body will be required to eliminate the excess nitrogen. Some experts believe this taxes the kidneys, and is one reason for an alarming increase in kidney trouble as people age. While more research is necessary, the evidence seems convincing and is one more reason why you don't need excess protein.

## Protein Need: Back to the RDI

Our protein needs vary with age. Growing children need more protein per pound of body weight than does an adult. On this body-weight basis, protein need declines to about age 20; after which it remains the same until our golden years, when it seems to increase again. For example, an infant requires 2.2 grams of protein per kilogram of body weight and an adult requires 0.8 grams per kilogram. Let me put that in perspective; imagine a 100-pound infant. The 100-pound infant would require 100 grams of protein; or 3.6 ounces daily. In contrast, a 100-pound adult requires 36 grams—that's only 1.28 ounces. An infant is a small metabolic dynamo because it's growing; in contrast, the adult's metabolism has slowed down to a maintenance program. Since infants are so small, they get along on less total protein, but if we fed them on a per-pound basis, we'd realize they require enormous amounts of food.

I've prepared Table 19.1 to show weight in pounds and kilograms, and the protein requirement in grams and ounces. This tabulation expresses the protein requirement of adults when the protein is of "good" quality but not "excellent," like casein or other animal protein, such as eggs, meat, or fish. You can see why the 65-gram requirement, expressed on many food labels, strikes a convenient average. If your protein is generally better than casein in quality, you can get by with less.

## TABLE 19.1

### Adult Protein Requirement

| Body Weight | | Protein Requirement | |
| --- | --- | --- | --- |
| Pounds | Kilograms | Grams | Ounces |
| 100 | 45 | 36 | 1.3 |
| 120 | 54 | 43 | 1.5 |
| 140 | 64 | 51 | 1.8 |
| 160 | 73 | 58 | 2.1 |
| 180 | 82 | 66 | 2.4 |
| 200 | 91 | 73 | 2.6 |

## The Caloric Cost of Protein Sources

Animal protein comes with the energy reserves animals store best—fat. Vegetable protein comes with carbohydrate, because that's how vegetables store energy. Since protein also provides calories, the total caloric delivery of food is a combination of protein, fat, and carbohydrate.

Table 19.2 (on the next two pages) illustrates how many calories are required to get an ounce (28 grams) of protein, or 43 percent of the recommended daily intake (RDI).

## TABLE 19.2

### The Caloric Costs of an Ounce of Protein

| Food | Amount in Ounces | Total Calories | Calories % as Fat | % as Carbohydrate |
|---|---|---|---|---|
| *Vegetable Foods* | | | | |
| Oatmeal (dry) | 6 (2 cups) | 663 | 16 | 68 |
| Soy beverage | 56 | 630 | 22 | 67 |
| Vegetable burgers | 4.9 | 217 | 4 | 23 |
| Vegetable sausage | 5.6 | 210 | 20 | 13 |
| Spaghetti | 26 (5.4 cups cooked) | 856 | 4 | 85 |
| Beans (baked, with pork) | 2 cups | 764 | 31 | 57 |
| Black beans* (boiled) | 1.8 cups | 418 | 4 | 72 |
| Mushrooms | 46 | 345 | 17 | 76 |
| White rice | 51 (7 cups) | 1,561 | None | 89 |
| Brown rice | 40 (5.7 cups) | 1,326 | 5 | 86 |
| Almonds | 4.7 | 821 | 75 | 12 |
| *Dairy Products* | | | | |
| Low fat 1% milk, protein fortified | 23 | 343 | 22 | 46 |
| Lactaid milk (low fat) | 28 | 357 | 26 | 47 |
| Yogurt (low fat) | 21 | 798 | 15 | 71 |
| Yogurt (cream) | 22 | 1,032 | 35 | 54 |
| Brick cheese | 4.2 | 445 | 72 | 3 |
| Cottage cheese (2% fat) | 7.3 | 182 | 20 | 16 |
| Egg | 8 (4.6 eggs) | 363 | 64 | 3 |

*Same for kidney beans, lima beans, and most other common beans.

| Food | Amount in Ounces | Total Calories | Calories | |
|------|------------------|----------------|----------|---|
| | | | % as Fat | % as Carbohydrate |

### Fish

| Food | Amount in Ounces | Total Calories | % as Fat | % as Carbohydrate |
|------|------------------|----------------|----------|-------------------|
| Striped bass | 5.6 | 152 | 22 | None |
| Salmon | 5.0 | 200 | 40 | None |

### Meat

| Food | Amount in Ounces | Total Calories | % as Fat | % as Carbohydrate |
|------|------------------|----------------|----------|-------------------|
| Regular ground beef | 4.3 | 349 | 66 | None |
| Prime rib | 4.5 | 471 | 75 | None |
| Bacon | 3.2 | 530 | 77 | None |
| Roast pork | 5.7 | 464 | 74 | None |
| Link sausage | 139 (11 links) | 516 | 77 | None |
| Beef frankfurter | 8.3 (4 franks) | 730 | 81 | 2 |

### Poultry

| Food | Amount in Ounces | Total Calories | % as Fat | % as Carbohydrate |
|------|------------------|----------------|----------|-------------------|
| Chicken, dark meat (no skin) | 3.5 | 205 | 42 | None |
| Chicken, white meat (no skin) | 3.2 | 157 | 23 | None |
| Turkey, white meat (no skin) | 3.3 | 147 | 18 | None |

Regarding the amount of specific foods required to get 1 ounce of protein: the data are for foods cooked without adding anything; for example, roasting meat, fish, or fowl, and boiling vegetables. The data are adopted from *Bowes and Church's Food Values of Portions Commonly Used,* by Jean A. Pennington (15th edition, 1989, J. B. Lippincott Co.), and from labels on standard products.

Table 19.2 shows that animal foods are the most efficient sources of protein. Compare, for example, fish, fowl, and lean meat to rice. To get adequate protein from rice would mean a lot of eating—as well as many calories. The most calorie-efficient protein sources are fish and the white meat of fowl.

Now focus your attention on soy sausage links and soy "hamburgers." These products, sold in the frozen section of supermarkets, are excellent protein sources with a low-fat cost.

Table 19.3 tabulates the protein in a typical day's meals. This simple food pattern contains 66 grams of protein from less than 1,000 calories, leaving room for other foods, desserts, snacks, flax oil, and fish oil capsules.

In addition to the protein sources in Table 19.3, you need at least two pieces of fruit, three vegetables, and one serving of beans. (An apple, pear, orange, or banana each counts as one fruit. A serving of vegetables would be spinach, carrots, or peas, to name just a few.)

## Table 19.3

### A Menu That Provides the RDI for Protein Under 1,000 Calories*

| Food | Serving Size | Protein (grams) | Calories |
|------|--------------|-----------------|----------|
| Oatmeal | 1/3 cup (dry) | 5 | 109 |
| Soy beverage | 1 cup | 4 | 88 |
| Salmon | 3.5 oz | 20 | 140 |
| Rice | 1 cup | 4 | 223 |
| Spaghetti | 1 cup | 5 | 158 |
|   with chicken | | 28 | 157 |
| Totals | | 66 | 875 |

*If other foods are eaten, for example, some breads, vegetables, and fruit, they will provide a little protein as well. This would be an excellent day's protein for people with IBD.

## Putting It Together

Protein, essential for life and health, can be obtained from many foods. A person with IBD should focus on fish and fowl (the most effective sources), eggs, nonfat and low-fat dairy products, and new options in man-made vegetarian sources of protein. Such a plan will create an excellent protein, fat, and carbohydrate balance as well as optimize the effectiveness of the omega-3 oil supplements.

Indeed, if every family member eats according to the same plan, all will be healthier for it, since selection of these protein sources and eating an abundance of fruits and vegetables will reduce the risk of cancer and heart disease.

# CHAPTER 20

# *Dietary Fats and Oils*

In Chapter Nine we discussed fats and oils as they relate to inflammation, and you can refer back to the glossary in that chapter as you read this. My objective here is to help you find your way among the available fats and oils to help you keep your IBD in remission.

We're all familiar with fat. You know intuitively that some foods, like butter, are all fat; other foods, such as bacon, ham, and prime rib of beef, are high in fat; and still others, such as white turkey meat and fish, are low in fat. Confusion abounds about fat since people mistakenly think that margarine and light oil, such as corn oil, have fewer calories than butter or heavy oil even though they don't. Foods, such as margarine, are advertised as having "no cholesterol" even if they're all fat, and that seems to create the illusion of "low calorie."

Nutritionists recommend that no more than 30 percent of our calories should come from fat. They add that we should strive for a ratio of polyunsaturated fat to saturated fat of 1:1, with the majority of fat as monounsaturated. So you might ask: "What's a polyunsaturated fat, and what's a monounsaturated fat?" Now if that's not enough, individuals with IBD should strive for as much dietary omega-3 oils as possible. If you feel a little confused, you're not alone, so we'll sort it out here.

## Saturated Versus Unsaturated Fat

A stick of butter, a tub of margarine, a bottle of olive oil, and a bottle of corn oil are all fat and each one provides 9 calories per gram. That's 252 calories per ounce (28 grams per ounce), or 85 calories per tablespoon. Olive oil is much better than butter for everyone, and especially for people with IBD—and it also outshines the corn oil.

You're already familiar with the two major groups of fat, saturated and unsaturated, although you might not have thought of them that way. Saturated fat is hard at room temperature and unsaturated fat is liquid at room temperature. Your refrigerator and cupboard probably have some excellent examples of each.

Butter is all saturated fat. It's solid at a cool room temperature and softens at body temperature. In fact, that's why we call saturated fat "hard fat." The hard white fat around a piece of beef, pork, or ham is also saturated fat. Though it's harder to see, the fat that marbles a filet of beef or prime rib is similarly saturated. All animal fat is hard at room temperature and becomes soft to liquid at body temperature.

In contrast to saturated fat, unsaturated fat is liquid at a cool room temperature. Perhaps you have some corn oil, peanut oil, or olive oil in your cupboard or pantry. All are clear liquids or amber-clear at room temperature. If you have several types, notice that some oils look clearer than others. Look at some safflower oil the next time you're in the supermarket, and notice that it is almost water clear. That's because it's almost 100 percent polyunsaturated.

You see, no natural fat is 100 percent polyunsaturated (PUFA) or saturated (SFA). Even butter contains some PUFA and most PUFAs contain some SFA.

Now you can differentiate fats by observing whether or not they are liquid or solid at room temperature. If it's liquid, it's mostly unsaturated, and if it's solid, it's mostly saturated. By inspection you can tell that some unsaturated oils are more polyunsaturated by their clarity. You can do another test. Put some oils in the refrigerator for about a day and notice how some become cloudy while other stay clear; the cloudy oils have more saturated fat. The more polyunsaturated— "poly" meaning much—an oil, the less likely it will get cloudy.

## Saturated (SFA), Monounsaturated (MFA), Polyunsaturated (PUFA)

The terms *saturated* and *unsaturated* describe the actual chemical structure of a fat. In a saturated fat (SFA for short) the actual linkages holding the carbon atoms together are all used up; the term *saturated* means "no openings." In monounsaturated oils (MFA for short) one linkage is unused; there is one opening, hence *mono*, meaning one. Since "poly" means many, it follows that in polyunsaturated oils (PUFA) many spaces are left open. Now you know why oils are unsaturated and hard fats are saturated. The more unsaturated, the lighter the oil.

Olive oil is an excellent example of MFA. While liquid at room temperature, MFA oils tend to be amber and somewhat thick, so they flow more slowly than PUFAs.

Sunflower oil is an excellent PUFA oil. It's light and very fluid—much more fluid than olive oil. The more unsaturated these PUFA oils, the clearer and easier they flow. Safflower, the most unsaturated of all the oils, looks and flows like water.

Beef lard is an SFA. It's solid and hard at body temperature, like most animal fat. Common examples of SFA are beef and pork fat. "Hard fat" is a good description for them.

## Olive Oil Bread and Mt. Everest

In Mediterranean countries, especially Italy and Greece, bread was traditionally not buttered, and still is not in many places. A small amount of olive oil was poured onto a plate and the bread dipped into the oil. Since olive oil is an MFA, it is much healthier than butter, does not contribute to heart disease, and actually reduces cancer risk. This "olive oil dipping" tradition is an example of how eating habits that promote health become established.

Mt. Everest climbers are faced with the problem of carrying sufficient calories up the mountain. A group of scientists under my direction, working on the nutritional requirements of this expedition, solved the problem by packing olive oil capsules that climbers learned to swallow with little or no water. Olive oil is fat, nature's most concentrated calorie source, and is the healthiest oil for the purpose. Our objective was to have the climbers reach the summit with a minimum loss in body weight. The olive oil capsules were so successful toward this goal that the tradition has been carried on in successive Mt. Everest expeditions.

## Omega-3 Versus Omega-6 Oils

Chemists can separate PUFAs even more based on the location of the open spaces in the fat molecules. Counting from one end of the fat molecule, called the omega end (the other is called the alpha end) of the fat molecule, the reactive center is either six units in, or three units in; so it's called either omega-6 or omega-3.

In North America our diets are rich in the omega-6 oils, which are found in abundance in corn, soy, and sunflower oils, and in animal fat—in short, everywhere. So when you eat baked goods, you are almost always getting a good helping of omega-6 oil—and in some foods, especially some pizza crusts, lard is actually used.

In contrast, the omega-3 oils are found in the chloroplasts of green plants, cold-water blue-skinned fish, nuts that grow on trees, and some seeds, such as flax, sesame, and several others. Since domesticated animals are fattened on corn, their fat reserves are omega-6. Omega-3 oils are only found in the fat of wild forage animals including deer, elk, moose, rabbit, and a few others most of us don't eat.

We could never eat enough green leafy vegetables to satisfy our need for omega-3 oils. Hence we need to get them from cold-water fish, such as salmon, mackerel, and anchovies, which either eat seaweed or algae containing lots of the omega-3 oils, or eat smaller fish that have eaten these plants.

## Sources of Dietary Fat

Table 20.1 (on page 214) lists food by the percent of fat. It also gives the composition of SFA, MFA, and PUFA as a percent of the food. The numbers don't always add up to 100 percent because the foods contain traces of other fatty materials. Fats such as butter and oils contain some water and traces of other components. In addition, some information is lost in rounding off. However, Table 20.1 gives the information you need to select food on the basis of its fat content. It will help you select foods that have a modest to low fat composition. For example, in trying to reduce total animal fat, select fish and the white meat of fowl. We'll cover this in greater detail later. For now, let's look at the omega-3 and omega-6 oils and see what rules seem to apply.

# TABLE 20.1

## The Fat Content of Food
## (Percent by Weight)

| Food | Fat | SFA | MFA | PUFA | Calories as % Fat |
|---|---|---|---|---|---|
| Milk 2% | 2 | 1.2 | 0.8 | — | 3 |
| Milk, skim | Trace | — | — | — | — |
| Cheese (average) | 32 | 1 | 11 | 3 | 70 |
| Ice cream (average) | 11 | 6 | 3 | 2 | 49 |
| Yogurt (low fat) | 2 | 1 | 1 | — | 29 |
| Egg | 12 | 4 | 6 | Trace | 67 |
| Beef (regular ground) | 20 | 10 | 10 | — | 62 |
| Beef (lean) | 20 | 9 | 9 | 2 | 62 |
| Chicken w/o skin | 3.5 | 1 | 1 | 1 | 23 |
| Chicken with skin | 6.5 | 2 | 3 | 2 | 29 |
| Chicken dark | 10 | 3 | 5 | 2 | 40 |
| Lamb (lean) | 8 | 4 | 3 | 1 | 38 |
| Lamb (lean & fat, ground) | 29 | 16 | 11 | 2 | 74 |
| Pork (lean) | 13 | 4 | 6 | 3 | 70 |
| Pork, ground with fat | 29 | 12 | 14 | 3 | 73 |
| Frankfurter | 27 | 27 | — | — | 79 |
| Shellfish | 2 | — | — | — | 14 |
| Finfish (oily) | 6 | — | 3 | 3 | 37 |
| Finfish (fillet) | 5 | None | 3 | 2 | 26 |
| Wheat bread | 2 | — | 2 | — | 10 |
| Chocolate cake with icing | 11 | 4 | 5 | 2 | 27 |
| Danish pastry | 22 | 7 | 11 | 4 | 50 |
| Beans (average) | None | None | — | — | None |
| Butter | 81 | 45 | 27 | 3 | 100 |
| Lard | 100 | 38 | 46 | 16 | 100 |
| Margarine | 81 | 15 | 41 | 22 | 100 |
| Corn oil | 100 | 10 | 28 | 53 | 100 |
| Cottonseed | 100 | 25 | 21 | 50 | 100 |
| Olive | 100 | 11 | 76 | 7 | 100 |
| Peanut | 100 | 18 | 47 | 29 | 100 |
| Safflower | 100 | 8 | 17 | 75 | 100 |
| Soybean | 100 | 15 | 20 | 52 | 100 |

Tables 20.2 and 20.3 list sources of omega-3 oils and the calorie content of commonly used spreads and oils. This information, along with Table 20.1, can be used to increase consumption of omega-3 oils and reduce total fat.

## TABLE 20.2

### Sources of Omega-3 Oils

| Food | Omega-3 Content<br>*(Grams per 3½-ounce Serving)* |
|------|---------------------------------------------------|
| Salmon | 1.0–2.6 |
| Mackerel | 0.7–2.6 |
| Anchovy | 0.7–1.5 |
| Cod | 0.3 |
| Striped bass | 0.2–0.8 |
| Snapper | 0.1–0.3 |
| Shellfish | 0.5 |
| Trout | 0.2–1.0 |
| Tuna | 0.4–2.5 |

### *Oils That Provide Omega-3 Oils*

| | |
|------|------|
| Walnut | Rapeseed |
| Flaxseed | Avocado |
| Sesame seed | Puritan oil |
| Soybean | Canola |
| Cod liver | |
| Salmon | |
| Menhaden | |

## TABLE 20.3

### Calorie Content of Commonly Used Spreads and Oils per Tablespoon

| Spreads | Calories |
|---------|----------|
| Butter | 108 |
| Whipped butter | 81 |
| Butter Buds (liquid) | 6 |
| Margarine (all sources) | 100 |
| Whipped margarine (all sources) | 70 |
| Diet margarine (low calorie) | 50 |

| Spreads | Calories |
|---|---|
| Mayonnaise | 100 |
| Low-calorie mayonnaise | 35 |
| Vegetable oil spreads | 80 |

## Cholesterol

Cholesterol is one of the buzzwords that characterize our society. Blood cholesterol is used as a simple index of our tendency to develop heart disease. As your blood cholesterol goes up, so does the sludge, called plaque, that gets deposited on the walls of your arteries, for among other things, plaque consists of cholesterol. It follows that we want to lower blood cholesterol.

Lowering cholesterol, or not letting it rise in the first place, means following four simple dietary rules:

1. Keep dietary cholesterol below 250 milligrams daily.
2. Eat a moderately low-fat diet, increase dietary PUFA, and avoid SFA.
3. Eat a high-fiber diet.
4. Maintain ideal weight. (This usually isn't a problem for people with IBD.)

Cholesterol is an animal product. Our bodies produce it because it's necessary for many functions, especially vitamin D production. There simply isn't any cholesterol in vegetable foods. So a margarine advertisement saying "No cholesterol" is like saying "Water is wet." It follows that we get cholesterol when we eat meat, dairy products, fish, or the flesh from anything that is not from the plant kingdom.

However, the major dietary sources of cholesterol are organ and high-fat meats. Look again at Table 20.1. As the percentage of saturated fat increases in animal food, so does the cholesterol content. Select low-fat meat, emphasize the white meat of fowl, and eat lots of fish. If you do, you'll keep your fat below 30 percent of calories and your cholesterol to less than 150 milligrams daily.

## Eggs Are Okay

Before I leave the discussion of cholesterol I must touch on the much-maligned egg. Eggs are good food! They provide the very best quality protein nature has to offer, and for the protein you get, eggs are inexpensive! In addition, eggs contain natural chemicals that help to lower blood cholesterol. The egg has simply gotten bad press; used in moderation, they're just about the best source of protein available in the supermarket. Moreover, the versatility of eggs in cooking is almost legend. But one large egg contains about 200 milligrams of cholesterol. Eating eggs a couple of times a week is fine, if you watch your cholesterol intake the rest of the time. If you follow the dietary advice in Part II, you will have no problem.

## Lecithin

Lecithin is a naturally occurring fat found in oil-bearing plants, egg yolks, and some animal fats. It has been credited with accomplishing everything from cholesterol reduction to improving mental abilities, so it seems worthwhile to discuss what lecithin actually *does* accomplish.

Lecithin consists of three major fatty substances: choline, inositol, and linoleic acid. You've already encountered linoleic acid. It's the major omega-6 PUFA found in plants with a moderate cholesterol-lowering ability. Choline and inositol are important for the function of your nervous system. At one time some scientists proposed that they be given the status of B vitamins, but this proposal was dropped. Still, the notion that they are vitamins persists, and you sometimes see them listed on vitamin preparations. Indeed, research has shown that they do help mental and nervous system function under some specialized conditions. This research was conducted using highly concentrated lecithin supplements that aren't available to the public; hence, the conclusion that lecithin improves mental acuity is correct, but not something the average person can accomplish with supplements.

The rumor that lecithin will dissolve fat, specifically cellulite, is complete nonsense. In fact, one could argue that using large amounts of lecithin could add to your fat and cellulite because it provides calories.

Should you use supplemental lecithin? In my opinion, our food provides all the lecithin we need. A person with IBD should use sensible food supplements that help provide a good balance of vitamins, minerals, fiber, and the omega-3 oils. I would prefer that you apply money spent on lecithin to more omega-3 oil supplements.

## Calories

Fats and oils in any form provide 9 calories per gram. No matter how important the product sounds, the calorie delivery is the same. The commonly used units of measure are listed in Table 20.4.

### TABLE 20.4

**Fat Calories in Some
Common Units of Measure**

| Unit | Calories |
|------|----------|
| *Weight* | |
| Gram | 9 |
| Ounce (28.35 grams) | 255 |
| Pound (454 grams) | 4,086 |
| *Volume* | |
| Teaspoon (4.9 ml, about 4.9 grams) | 44 |
| Tablespoon (3 teaspoons) | 133 |
| 1 fluid ounce (2 tablespoons) | 266 |
| 1 cup (8 fluid ounces) | 2,129 |

Whenever you put a 1-ounce pat of butter on a baked potato, stop and think about this: A baked potato provides
about 200 calories depending on size; 1 ounce of butter or
margarine adds 255 calories. Put another way, the condiment
contributes more calories than the food! Potatoes by themselves are not fattening. Sour cream has half the calories of
butter, and have you ever tried a baked potato with olive oil?

What about low-calorie spreads? All spreads contain varying levels of fat. Some contain water; some are whipped and
contain air; still others are blended with starch and contain
fewer calories. I've listed some commonly used spreads to
give you a feeling for the calories per serving.

From Table 20.3 you can see that most spreads that look,
act, and feel like butter deliver about 100 calories per tablespoon. Whipping and reducing the oil or fat by about 50 percent reduces calories to about 50 per tablespoon. Butter
Buds are a truly low-calorie substitute for butter.

## Get Good Fat Balance: Putting It All Together

Fat is one of the most important and least understood elements of your diet. Now that we've explored the types of dietary fat that we get from food, we'll learn how we should put
them together in a good diet. First a few rules.

*Rule 1:* Keep fat to fewer than 30 percent of calories.
*Rule 2:* Maintain as little SFA as possible.
*Rule 3:* PUFA should be about 6 percent of calories.
*Rule 4:* Keep cholesterol below about 250 milligrams daily.
*Rule 5:* Strive for omega-3 oils in foods, and use EPA sup-
plements and flax oil.

We'll discuss carbohydrates in the next chapter, but at this
point we can already plan a diet that delivers plenty of protein and only 30 percent of calories from fat. I'll give you
some do's and don'ts that work.

## Dietary Do's

*Do* eat red meat only once monthly.

*Do* select white meat from fish or poultry.

*Do* eat an egg twice weekly.

*Do* use olive oil for cooking.

*Do* learn to use olive oil as a spread.

*Do* eat fish four times weekly.

*Do* use alternates to butter, such as sour cream on potatoes.

*Do* select nonfat dairy products.

## Don'ts

*Don't* eat processed meats.

*Don't* eat cheese more than twice weekly.

*Don't* eat organ meats.

*Don't* eat the skin on fowl.

*Don't* use butter.

*Don't* eat eggs more than twice weekly.

*Don't* cook food in butter, lard, or other saturated fat.

*Don't* use whole milk.

# CHAPTER 21

# Carbohydrates: First Fuel

Your body has an elaborate system to maintain a constant blood glucose level, and about 3 percent of your body weight is a reserve carbohydrate, glycogen, found in your organs and tissues. Circulating blood glucose is available instantly, and glycogen can be mobilized in an instant to maintain blood levels; they are the first fuel sources the body calls on. So, when you run up the stairs, do a 100-yard dash, or do some mental gymnastics, such as jump to conclusions, the energy comes from blood glucose, which is quickly replenished from your glycogen reserves.

The reason you're out of breath after running up stairs is because you burned the glucose a little faster than your lungs could supply the necessary oxygen, so you're simply repaying that oxygen debt until your metabolism catches up and restores balance. You would have had to keep jogging about fifteen minutes before your body would start mobilizing your fat reserves.

Your brain uses about 20 percent of your circulating blood glucose—there is no analogy to the 100-yard dash—so you can't use mental energy fast enough to create an oxygen debt. In contrast, your brain responds quickly when blood glucose drops significantly with various emotional responses that alert you and send you in search of food.

These mental responses testify to the importance of blood glucose.

These insights indicate how important dietary carbohydrates are to your health, so it's not surprising that carbohydrates are abundant in natural foods. Sometimes it is to our detriment that it is abundant in man-made foods. In natural foods, carbohydrates are ideally suited for human health. In contrast, man-made foods seldom include ideal carbohydrates and thus are quite the opposite of natural foods.

## What Are Carbohydrates?

Carbohydrates contain carbon, hydrogen, and oxygen, the elements of water; hence, "hydrate." The two most ubiquitous carbohydrates are glucose and fructose, both found abundantly in nature. Other carbohydrates (except for one found in mother's milk) are made in plants of or from these two simple sugars. Not surprisingly, they have a common origin.

## Photosynthesis and Glucose and Fructose

Photosynthesis is the process in which a green plant uses sunlight energy to extract carbon dioxide from the air and combine it with water to make the simple sugar glucose. This exceedingly complex process is common to all plants and testifies to the importance of solar energy. When your body uses the energy in food, whether fat or carbohydrate, you are indirectly using solar energy. Glucose is the primary product of the conversion of solar energy to chemical energy, so it's most ubiquitous. Most animals, including humans, use glucose for physical and mental energy.

Living things, including humans, can rearrange glucose to make fructose, which is why it is as widely distributed as glucose, but in a little less quantity. Glucose and fructose are "monosaccharides" because they're single units; "mono" means one. And they're sweet; hence "saccharide."

Many plants can link glucose and fructose together to make sucrose, a disaccharide, which is common table sugar. Table sugar is the purest and cheapest organic chemical available worldwide. Two glucose units are often arranged into another disaccharide, called maltose. Maltose is found in germinating seeds, such as barley, wheat, and other seed grains.

Galactose is a fourth simple sugar with a slightly different structure than glucose. It is the only sugar made exclusively from glucose by animals. Galactose is linked with glucose to form lactose, a common disaccharide found in the milk of all mammals. So human infants share the same nutritional nurturing as other mammals.

## Sugar Alcohols

Plants can change glucose to a number of other simple, generally unimportant sugars, which include xylose, pentose, and sedoheptulose. Some of these sugars are converted by plants, or commercially, into sugar alcohols. Two of them, sorbitol and xylitol, made from sucrose and xylose, respectively, are sweet and widely used.

## Sweetness

We are born with the ability to detect sweet, sour, salty, and bitter tastes. Sweet detection was more important in early human history than it is now. This is because in nature, sweet things provide energy and are generally safe to eat; sour-tasting things are often spoiled and can contain harmful germs and cause illness; bitter foods often contain toxic, even addictive substances; and drinking salt water can kill anyone, especially an infant. Military Survival Schools teach men to eat sweet things and avoid bitter things for survival when trapped behind enemy lines.

Fructose, the sweetest sugar, is what makes fruits, berries, and some vegetables sweet. Sucrose, common table sugar, is next in sweetness; it gets its sweetness from the fructose it contains, rather than its glucose, which has only half the sweetness of fructose. Xylitol, a sugar alcohol, is about as sweet as sucrose, but is not widely used.

Table 21.1 summarizes the sweetness of the most common sugars and shows that after fructose and sucrose, there's no contest.

## Table 21.1

**Relative Sweetness of Common Sugars**

| Sugar | Relative Sweetness |
| --- | --- |
| Fructose | 1.0 |
| Sucrose | 0.8 |
| Glucose | 0.6 |
| Maltose | 0.3 |
| Lactose | 0.2 |
| *Sugar Alcohols* | |
| Xylitol | 0.8 |
| Sorbitol | 0.4 |

## Complex Carbohydrates: Starches

Glucose, fructose, and maltose, a disaccharide, can be linked together in almost endless chains called complex carbohydrates, or starches. In this case, "complex" simply means large.

Starch is stored by the plant as an energy source. That's why potatoes, rice, wheat, corn, turnips, beans, cereals, grains, and vegetables are starchy. They represent the storage of energy for reproduction. About 10,000 years ago, people discovered the food value of starch, and agriculture began. This led to farming of the major grains, cereals, tubers, beans, and other vegetable foods.

You might ask: "Why isn't an apple or pear starchy?" Apples, pears, cherries, and most fruits do contain starch, but in the seeds or pits, which we don't eat. For the seeds to be spread, and the species to survive, they rely on animals, even humans, to eat the fruit and either spit out the seeds or pass them in stools.

## Dietary Fiber

Some glucose and maltose are made into carbohydrate materials that resist digestion by most animals, including humans. These include cellulose, pectin, and a few other materials that we call dietary fiber. Dietary fiber is plant carbohydrate material that isn't digested. Chapter Sixteen is devoted to dietary fiber, but here I want you to see how it relates to carbohydrate metabolism.

Plant cells are protected by a cell wall that's made of tough, coarse fibers called cellulose. These cells are bound together with other nondigestible materials such as lignins, mucilage, and pectins. These materials give the plant its shape, protect fruit from drying out, hold parts of it together, and bind water. Fiber comes in many forms and serves many purposes. For humans, all fibers have one thing in common: they aren't digested by our digestive enzymes even though some dietary fiber is broken down by bacteria that inhabit the large intestine.

## Blood Glucose and Muscle Glycogen

Your blood contains, on average, 80 to 100 milligrams of glucose per 100 milliliters. We call it 80 to 100 milligram percent. We'll talk more about blood glucose later, but for now, recognize that it's the major, instant energy source for everything we do. Since this means glucose is also the brain's energy source, when it drops below 80, we become anxious.

Glycogen is a reserve carbohydrate, like starch, but glycogen's structure is like a netting rather than a chain. This netting can release many glucose units at once, so in times of emergency, glycogen disintegrates, pouring glucose into your blood, muscles, and organs, where it provides quick energy.

Glycogen is stored in your muscles, liver, kidneys, and other organs to be used as required. When your blood glucose is being used, such as during active exercise, glycogen is mobilized to keep your blood glucose up. When glycogen has been depleted, such as during long periods of activity, a starchy meal restores your glycogen reserves. That's why athletes train with large amounts of high-carbohydrate meals to build glycogen reserves.

## Carbohydrate as Energy

Carbohydrate provides 4 calories per gram, which is a little less than half of the calories of fat. This is because carbohydrates are halfway to the end products of energy production—they're about half-metabolized. Fat, on the other hand, isn't metabolized at all, so it has more energy.

When carbon materials yield their energy, two chemical by-products are given off: carbon dioxide and water. Oxygen is used for combustion, so when we completely burn gasoline, fat, paper, wood, or sugar—along with energy used or released as heat—the only by-products are carbon dioxide and water. When your body burns glucose or fat, it traps energy in other substances, maintaining a constant 98.6°F. The more efficient the engine, the cooler it runs, so your body is much more efficient than any engine. And you don't light up!

In contrast to fat that hasn't been metabolized at all, carbohydrate is more easily and more quickly metabolized to produce energy, and it only calls for half the oxygen of fat. Therefore, glucose is used for energy first because it's the best source. When the need is longer-term, such as in jogging, the body mobilizes its fat reserves and starts burning fat. This is easily seen by comparing the body's requirements for a 100-yard run to a 3-mile run.

A 100-yard run takes an average person less than a half minute. The body can supply the energy with its blood glucose; there's not even a need to mobilize glycogen. The 3-mile run, in contrast, will take the same person twenty-five minutes. After the first five minutes the body mobilizes its glycogen, and by ten minutes, it starts using the circulating blood fats. After fifteen minutes, as much as 50 percent of the energy for running comes from fat, and fat reserves are being called into action.

## Digestion of Carbohydrate

In the Preface you observed that digestion begins in the mouth with chewing and lubrication. Saliva, in addition to moistening and lubricating food, also contains an enzyme that breaks down starch. You can prove this to yourself by chewing a soda cracker, which is loaded with starch. You'll notice how it starts out bland and slowly begins to taste sweet. The starch in soda crackers breaks down in your mouth to maltose, which in Table 21.1 is shown as mildly sweet. However, very little metabolism of starch takes place in the mouth since the food is swallowed, and the saliva enzymes continue for a while in the stomach.

In the small intestine, starches are completely broken down to glucose; sucrose is broken into glucose and fructose. Lactose is split by the enzyme lactase into glucose and galactose. (The lack of lactase in some ethnic groups was discussed in Chapter Four.)

## Absorption of Sugar

Humans don't absorb starch into the blood; we only absorb the simple sugars glucose, fructose, and galactose, and a few other minor sugars and sugar alcohols.

Since starch is like a long chain and digestion proceeds from the ends, gluclose is released slowly from starch. We urge people to eat a diet rich in complex carbohydrates (starches) because glucose is released slowly into the blood as digestion proceeds down the intestine. That is why vegetables, grains, and cereals are so important.

In contrast to starch, when you eat food or drink a beverage that's rich in sucrose, the glucose is almost instantly ready for absorption. As soon as it enters the intestine, the glucose quickly crosses into the blood. This rapid sugar load, high in the intestine, signals the body to produce the hormone insulin, which allows the glucose in the blood to enter each cell.

A heavy sugar load elevates blood sugar and insulin production is excessive, so the glucose quickly enters the body cells and causes the blood glucose to drop quickly, producing low blood sugar, or hypoglycemia. "Hypo" means low and "glycemia" means sugar. The brain responds with anxiety, because if glucose gets too low, the brain can't function; you become anxious (to outsiders, irritable). The body mobilizes glycogen and the solution is to eat more food. It is one reason why these foods are fattening. You might ask: "What about fruits? They contain lots of sugars."

## Fiber in Absorption: Why Fruit Sugar Isn't the Same

Dietary fiber plays an important role in the absorption of glucose. A scientific experiment tells the fiber story very nicely.

The scientists used apples prepared in three ways: raw, pureed into an opaque juice with lots of pulp, and as a clarified juice by filtering the puree. Each preparation was adjusted so it provided the same amount of glucose and fructose as the apple. They had volunteers fast for twelve hours, then eat each of them. On each of three successive days the volunteers received a different preparation. In that way, each person served as his or her own control.

The apple, as the baseline, changed the blood sugar very little even though all the glucose and fructose from the apple was absorbed. The heavy puree raised blood sugar just under 10 percent from its fasting level. In contrast, the clarified juice (fiber removed) elevated the blood glucose by more than 20 percent. In each case insulin production was in proportion to the blood sugar change. Consequently, about ninety minutes after drinking the highly clarified juice, the volunteers had low blood sugar, and they were hungry. The only difference between each preparation was the fiber. The apple presented a matrix that consisted of fiber, especially pectin and cellulose. Although the matrix was destroyed in the thick puree, most of the fiber was still present. In the clarified juice there was no fiber.

Fiber modulates the absorption of sugar, so it is similar to eating starch. Actually, fiber modulates the absorption of fat and amino acids as well, but it's most important in the absorption of glucose and fructose. Therefore, even though it is not digested itself, fiber is an essential component in carbohydrate digestion and absorption.

## Protein and Carbohydrate Absorption

Protein-rich food also helps to modulate glucose and fructose absorption. This is because protein provides a complex mixture in the intestine, and since protein is digested slowly, the sugar is slowly released. Consequently, a protein-rich meal containing sugar-rich foods modulates sugar absorption. So, dessert following a meal doesn't produce a sugar "surge" in the blood like it would if it were eaten on an empty stomach.

## Selecting Carbohydrate-rich Foods

Eat natural foods, or starch-rich foods such as breads and pastas! Our food selections should emphasize fruits, vegetables, cereals, and grains. When selecting processed foods, choose pasta, cereals (such as Shredded Wheat), whole-grain breads, and foods made with whole potatoes and rice. The apple experiment teaches that juices made from whole fruit should always be selected.

Table 21.2 lists the carbohydrate content of some natural foods so you can get a feeling for the percentage of calories from carbohydrates. As you can see, most vegetables and fruits are principally carbohydrates. On average, more than 70 percent of their calories come from carbohydrates. Some fruits, such as oranges, are almost all carbohydrate. Nuts and avocados are exceptions, since their calories are largely derived from the oils they contain.

## Table 21.2

## Carbohydrate-rich Foods

| Food | Serving Size | Grams Carbohydrate | Calories | Carbohydrates as Percent Total Calories |
|---|---|---|---|---|
| Milk (2%) | 1 cup | 15 | 60 | 41 |
| Yogurt | 1 cup | 13 | 52 | 42 |
| Cheese | 1 oz | Trace | None | None |
| Nuts (average) | 1 cup | 28 | 96 | 11 |
| Beans and peas | 1 cup | 38 | 152 | 72 |
| Asparagus | 1 cup | 5 | 20 | 67 |
| Broccoli | 1 cup | 7 | 28 | 70 |
| Cauliflower | 1 cup | 5 | 20 | 80 |
| Potato, baked (no skin) | 1 potato | 21 | 84 | 93 |
| Potato, boiled (no skin) | 1 potato | 23 | 92 | 87 |
| Tomato | 1 cup | 10 | 40 | 80 |
| Avocado | 1 avocado | 13 | 52 | 14 |
| Banana | 1 banana | 26 | 104 | 100 |
| Grapefruit | 1/2 grapefruit | 12 | 48 | 100 |
| Orange | 1 orange | 16 | 64 | 100 |
| Apple | 1 apple | 18 | 72 | 85 |
| Apricots | 3 apricots | 14 | 56 | 100 |
| Raspberries | 1 cup | 17 | 68 | 97 |
| Bagel | 1 bagel | 30 | 120 | 73 |
| French bread | 1-pound loaf | 251 | 1,004 | 76 |
| Rye bread | 1 slice | 13 | 72 | 87 |
| White bread | 1 slice | 10 | 40 | 73 |
| Whole wheat bread | 1 slice | 14 | 56 | 86 |
| Cake with chocolate icing | 1 piece | 45 | 180 | 72 |
| Spaghetti (cooked) | 1 cup | 32 | 128 | 83 |
| Shredded Wheat | 1 biscuit | 20 | 80 | 88 |

Low-fat milk and yogurt provide about 42 percent of calories from carbohydrate and most of the remainder from protein. Cheese does not follow this pattern; it provides most of its calories from fat. Breads and other foods made from grains provide about 70 percent or more of their calories from carbohydrate.

From this analysis, you can get a feeling for carbohydrates as a percentage of the calories of most natural foods. But this leaves packaged and processed foods. You might ask, what about pizza? Breakfast cereals? How do you know which fruit juice to select? This requires label reading and we'll deal with that next.

## Label Reading for Carbohydrates

The nutritional panel on most products provides a complete breakdown of carbohydrates. The top of the nutrition panel shows total carbohydrate content per serving. Multiply this number by 4 to get the total calories from carbohydrate and divide it into total calories and multiply by 100 to get the percentage of calories from carbohydrate. Then, look at the bottom of the panel under *Total Carbohydrate Information,* which gives the breakdown of starch and related carbohydrates, and sucrose and other sugars, if they are present. Let's look at the ingredients list.

## Ingredients List

On the same panel that contains nutrition information is an ingredients list expressed in descending order by weight of the ingredients used to make the product. We'll use Product 19 as an example of readily available breakfast cereal.

Its ingredients list reads: corn, oat and wheat flour, sugar, rice, salt, defatted wheat germ, corn syrup, malt flavoring, annatto color. The information continues with a listing of added vitamins and minerals, which we'll cover later. Product 19's ingredients list tells you that this cereal is mostly starch and contains two sources of sugar: sugar (meaning table sugar) and corn syrup (which is mostly fructose and glucose).

From the ingredients list and nutrition label of Product 19

you can also conclude that the cereal is mostly starch, with very little whole grain, because 83 percent—20 of the 24 grams of carbohydrate—is starch. Another 13 percent is sugar, so that leaves little room for fiber. A cereal providing less than 3 grams of fiber per serving is not a whole-grain cereal!

The uppermost part of the nutrition panel states that the cereal provides 24 grams of carbohydrate per serving. Four times 24, divided into 100 (total calories per serving) and multiplied by 100 tells you that 96 percent of the calories in this product come from carbohydrates.

Now go to the bottom of the panel under *Carbohydrate Information*. First, it tells you that starch and related carbohydrates are 20 grams; that means 20 of 24 grams of complex carbohydrate. Next it states that it contains 3 grams of sucrose and other sugars; meaning about 13 percent of the carbohydrate is simple sugar. Product 19 provides 1 gram of fiber, which is not enough.

Two comparisons to Product 19 are Nabisco Shredded Wheat and Quaker Oats. I'll leave their nutritional panels for you to read the next time you're in the supermarket.

Nabisco Shredded Wheat has a simple ingredients list. Ingredients: "100% natural whole wheat." It's clean—no sugar, no oils, nothing added. Quaker Oats is a cooked cereal that provides an ideal type of fiber for everybody, especially people with bowel disorders. (I recommend you make it without salt.) It too is an elegantly simple cereal. Ingredients: "100% natural rolled oats."

I'll give you one last comparison: the ingredients list for Cap'n Crunch. It speaks for itself; the product is flour, white and brown sugar, and sprayed-on vitamins, some of which are used in lesser quantity than the product's artificial color:

*Ingredients:* Corn flour, sugar, oat flour, coconut oil, brown sugar, salt, niacinamide [one of the B vitamins], reduced iron, yellow 5, calcium pantothenate [one of the B vitamins], zinc oxide [a source of zinc], yellow 6, pyridoxine hydrochloride [one of the B vitamins], thiamin mononitrate, BHA [a preservative], riboflavin, folic acid, vitamin B₁.

The lesson here is that sugar is sugar whether it's white or brown. Since corn flour contains some sugar, this product probably contains more sugar than any other ingredient. Another red flag is a sixth ingredient, salt, which we'll discuss in Chapter Twenty-three.

## Juice

I picked two fruit juices purchased in our local Safeway, for which we only need to read the ingredients list. The nutritional panel will tell you that they provide all their calories from carbohydrates and all the carbohydrates are in the form of simple sugar. However, the ingredients list can be very revealing.

### Hawaiian Punch
*Ingredients:* HP water, corn syrup and sugar, fruit juices and purees, concentrated pineapple, passion fruit, orange and grapefruit juices, apricot, papaya and guava purees, citric acid [provides tartness], natural flavors, vitamin C, dextrin [a flavor carrier], artificial color, artificial flavor, ethyl maltol [a flavor enhancer].

### Tiaman's Original Apple Juice
*Ingredients:* Made from Anderson Valley's finest apples; all natural—no additives, no concentrates.

Hawaiian Punch is mostly water; the HP simply means it's highly purified. That's good. The next two ingredients are sugar. Corn syrup is sugar and added to sugar makes this product mostly water and sugar. After that comes a number of fruit concentrates, followed by flavors and flavor enhancers. Since artificial and natural flavors have been added, it's obvious that the juice extracts aren't strong enough to flavor the sugar water.

Hawaiian Punch is really artificially flavored and colored sugar water. Do you want to put this into your body? In comparison, the Tiaman's Original Apple Juice is simply apple juice. It's cloudy, so it's got apple pulp. The pulp settles to some extent, so it needs to be shaken before being used. But it's quite close to an apple puree. It's a good product and makes an excellent beverage.

From the ingredients list and the nutritional label you can learn much about the source and type of carbohydrates in packaged foods. More than that, the ingredients list tells you how a product has been made. Using both panels regularly and correctly can help you make wise food selections. A good question to ask yourself after analyzing both lists is: "Do I want to put these ingredients into my body?"

## "Do's" and "Don'ts" for Carbohydrates

Carbohydrate-rich foods should make up about 50 to 60 percent of calories in your regular diet. However, selection should emphasize foods rich in complex carbohydrate and not simple sugar, with the exception of fruit, which is naturally balanced with a fiber to modulate its sugar absorption.

---

### Carbohydrate Do's

*Do* eat at least one serving of whole-grain cereal each day. Select ones that don't irritate your intestinal tract.

*Do* eat at least two fruit servings daily, such as an apple, pear, banana, or three apricots, or alternatively, a full cup of berries, if they do not cause intestinal irritation. Fruit should be peeled; canned fruit can also be used.

*Do* eat at least two servings of vegetables, such as asparagus, broccoli, spinach, or brussels sprouts.

*Do* eat at least one serving daily of a starchy vegetable, such as potatoes, rice, squash, or pasta.

*Do* eat one serving of some beans or other legumes.

---

These include kidney, pinto, navy and lima beans, to name only a very few.

*Do* eat one serving of salad with generous green leafy vegetables and aim for a colored vegetable such as red peppers, tomatoes, or carrots.

*Do* eat at least one serving of whole-grain bread, including wheat, rye, or another type, such as oat bread.

*Do* drink fruit juice that is made from natural fruit and is, at most, partially clarified. Read the ingredients list.

### Don'ts

*Don't* eat packaged foods in which sugar is one of the first two ingredients.

*Don't* drink juices that contain sugar or corn syrup, especially those with both.

*Don't* select breakfast cereals that provide fewer than 3 grams of dietary fiber in a 1-cup serving.

*Don't* drink more than one serving of sugar-containing soft drinks daily.

*Don't* use spreads that contain sugar except for a condiment such as catsup or mustard.

*Don't* use sugar except with a fiber-rich food, such as cereal, or as an accompaniment to a fiber-rich meal, such as in a cup of tea or coffee.

# CHAPTER 22

# *Calcium: A Case for Strong Bones*

It bears repeating that calcium is a difficult nutrient for most people, let alone anyone who has intestinal problems. It is probably the only nutrient for which shortfalls are additive. If you fall short for a year or two when you're a teenager, and then fall short again during your childbearing years, you will have less dense bones than if you hadn't fallen short at all. You would show no outward signs unless your density was very low, in which case low back pain might occur. Below-normal bone density is a disease called osteoporosis, which causes much suffering and even death in old age.

As with most nutrients, calcium is probably most critical for small children and through the teenage years. However, it is still extremely important throughout life. Calcium shortfalls affect women most because of childbearing and nursing, followed later by menopause. For those reasons, our discussion focuses mostly on women; however, it is also an important nutrient for men at all ages, especially after they enter life's sixth decade.

After age 10, girls need 1,000 milligrams of calcium daily, which continues into adulthood up to about age 50; after that, most nutritionists believe that calcium intake should be elevated to 1,500 milligrams, and many even recommend 2,000 milligrams daily. Most people, especially people with

IBD, cannot consume sufficient dairy products and calcium-rich foods each day. So, common sense says to use calcium supplements (up to about 1,000 milligrams of calcium daily)—and that's what most experts do.

## 1,000 Milligrams of Calcium from Common Foods

| Food | Amount | Calories | Comments |
|---|---|---|---|
| Cheddar cheese | 5.0 oz | 560 | Fat is bad |
| Low-fat cottage cheese | 5.2 oz | 1,066 | Too much fat and sodium |
| Skim milk | 27 fl oz (3⅓ 8-oz glasses) | 290 | Good source |
| Low-fat yogurt | 19 oz | 466 | Good source |
| Fortified orange juice | 27 fl oz (3⅓ 8-oz glasses) | 400 | Excellent source High potassium |

Most government nutrition and food analyses prove that calcium is generally short in most people's diets. In fact, many experts both use and recommend calcium supplements. In addition to the difficulty of obtaining adequate dietary calcium, many lifestyle habits, such as caffeine use, excess sodium intake, and lack of exercise, cause calcium loss; and it follows that these people need more calcium to compensate for such loss. Therefore, common sense dictates taking at least 600 milligrams of calcium daily—as nutrition insurance. Indeed, IBD patients could do better by taking 1,000 to 1,200 milligrams of calcium as supplements.

Bone calcium loss is accelerated by caffeine (coffee, tea, soft drinks), excess meat, salt, and inadequate exercise. However, much clinical research in many countries and across ethnic lines has proven that bone density can be restored by using calcium supplements. If you drink more than 2 cups of coffee or its equivalent as tea or soft drinks (10 cups or cans), take an extra 200 milligrams daily. Exercise is essential no matter how much calcium you take. The old saying "if you don't use it, you lose it" applies to bones.

## Magnesium: A Partner with Calcium

Most dietary analyses indicate that we usually also fall short in the mineral magnesium. Since 200 to 400 milligrams of magnesium are required daily, it, like calcium, cannot possibly fit into two multiple-vitamin tablets. Therefore, since you must take calcium as a separate supplement, take one that also contains some magnesium.

Some self-proclaimed experts advise a specific calcium-magnesium ratio for good health. Dr. Mildred Seelig conducted a careful study of adult needs for calcium and magnesium and proved that once you take in about 400 milligrams of magnesium daily, the body can use calcium very effectively, and there is no need to get more magnesium.

## Calcium Supplements

Selecting a calcium supplement is not difficult, so I've provided some points to follow:

- Choose a supplement that supplies 150 to 350 milligrams of calcium per tablet. It should also contain magnesium, another mineral that's usually deficient when your calcium level is low.
- Don't take more than about 400 milligrams of calcium as a supplement at a single meal. For if you take too much at one time, you won't absorb up to 35 percent; and you'll probably absorb only about 15 percent. Absorption of any nutrient is less efficient when there's too much.
- Take calcium supplements at mealtime because food, especially carbohydrates, helps with calcium absorption.
- Much research supports calcium citrate as an ideal supplement.

## Calcium from Food

Getting enough calcium from food isn't difficult, but it requires care:

- *Milk:* Use 8 ounces of low-fat milk on cereal every day.
- *Dairy products:* Select low-fat yogurt or cheese regularly.
- *Vegetables:* Select dark green ones. Take an extra serving, as the calories are insignificant and the nutritional value outstanding.
- *Snacks:* Use hard cheese sparingly. One ounce of hard cheese goes a long way.
- *Fortified foods:* Calcium-fortified foods, such as orange juice, are practical.

Bone density can be routinely and painlessly measured in all women. It should be done before menopause, say around age 45, and about three years after menopause. The objective is to enter menopause with good bone density and maintain it thereafter. All women and men need calcium, and I believe they need calcium supplements as well. However, some postmenopausal women also need supplemental estrogen as determined by bone density measurements.

You'd think that it would be good news if your doctor said your bone density is 25 percent or 50 percent above average. It is except for one point: bone density depends on calcium, exercise, and estrogen. So if your bone density is above average, you get 1,200 milligrams of calcium daily, and exercise vigorously regularly, you're in safe territory.

## Another Misconception Falls:
## Kidney Stones

Using calcium supplements always raises the question "Does extra calcium cause kidney stones?" This question comes up because most kidney stones contain calcium, and many doctors tell people who have kidney stones to avoid calcium. Those doctors are wrong!

Kidney stones in men and women are not caused by excess or even normal levels of calcium. If anything, careful studies show that extra calcium, even taken as a supplement, reduces the risk of kidney stones. The research clearly proves extra calcium does not cause kidney stones.

If you have a tendency to form kidney stones, you can do several things to prevent them—drink lots of water and orange juice, eat more fruits and vegetables, eat more foods rich in magnesium, and avoid grapefruit and grapefruit juice.

## When Should People Begin Calcium Supplementation?

Dietary study after dietary study indicates that most women and men begin falling short in calcium around the age they start using soft drinks and eating hamburgers—the teenage years.

Similarly, studies have shown that sensible calcium supplements help women enter adulthood with stronger, more dense bones, and that this strength prevails during childbearing years into the forties. Emphasis is on "sensible" once again.

Taking an extra 600 to 1,000 milligrams of calcium daily as a supplement (which will put your daily total calcium level in the safe and effective range of 1,000 to 1,400 milligrams) will pay big dividends throughout life.

# CHAPTER 23

# *Potassium and Sodium*

The diarrhea associated with IBD causes potassium loss. If you couple this with a diet of processed foods high in sodium, then add the side effects of medication, you've got a recipe for electrolyte imbalance. Over the years, such an imbalance can lead to high blood pressure. The objective of this chapter is to motivate you to prevent all those problems by sensible food selection.

## Critical Electrolyte Balance

When you look in the mirror it is hard to believe you're about 75 percent water. In fact, you could crudely describe humans as about 35 trillion cells (that's 35 followed by 12 zeros) that are mostly water, floating in a well-shaped sack of water. With all that water, it is a wonder that every body function is controlled by electrical currents that pass through nerves and muscle fibers. How does electricity move in all that water? And with such order and precision?

Fluid balance and nerve impulse transmission is so complex that it fills volumes. But in very simple terms, it depends on a critical balance of two electrolytes inside and outside of each cell, especially the nerve cells. The two principal electrolytes are sodium and potassium, with secondary involvement from calcium, magnesium, and a few other trace minerals. Sodium and potassium each carry a positive charge that is largely, but not completely, balanced by chloride, which has a negative charge.

Think of it: your body is constantly becoming aware of the environment with sight, sound, feel, and smell, to name four senses, and controlling your heart rate, muscle movement, and myriad other processes all at once. It is a far more complex control system than the computers that guide rocket liftoffs at Cape Kennedy. But without the correct balance of sodium and potassium inside and outside of each cell, your body would go awry, and if you survived at all, the effects on your health would be disastrous.

When the balance goes wrong—and it usually does so slowly—insidious problems, such as high blood pressure, arise. However, when it goes wrong quickly, dehydration often results that can causes fatigue, confusion, and at its worst, a stroke or heart attack.

## A Critical Ratio

Analyze any person, dog, cow, or other animal, and you'd find he or she consists of at least three times as much potassium as sodium. This ratio of just over 3 to 1 is consistent throughout the animal kingdom, because for any living body to function correctly, the same functions are essential. In fact, we each have an elaborate system to maintain this crucial balance directed by the kidneys, with secondary involvement by the taste buds and sweat glands. This balance is so critical that we each have two kidneys, even though just one can handle the job. When a back-up system exists, we call it redundancy, meaning that nature has endowed us with extra capacity in case one fails, or for an emergency to restore balance quickly.

The reason we don't have two hearts or brains is that the extra lung and kidney capacity is expected to protect those two vital organs against emergencies. This allows us to live out our life expectancy potential, which most experts place between 120 and 150 years.

## K-Factor

*K-factor* is the name we give to the dietary ratio of potassium to sodium. In natural foods, the K-factor is usually 3 or more (3 parts potassium to 1 part sodium). Natural diets usually have a K-factor above 5, because most natural foods have a K-factor over 10, and many vegetables are over 100. When the dietary K-factor among people falls to 1 (equal amounts of sodium and potassium), about 23 percent of adults and 5 percent of children will get high blood pressure. Modern diets now stand at a K-factor of 0.83, and high blood pressure is our most widespread health problem even though you don't hear about it very often. The K-factor declines because of widespread use of processed foods and too much salt in home- and restaurant-cooked natural foods.

## Examples of K-Factors

The K-factor is obtained by taking the ratio of potassium to sodium in food. Once you get the knack, it's easy. Table 23.1 compares some natural foods with their processed counterparts. Notice that natural foods are low in sodium and have an excellent K- factor.

### Table 23.1

#### K-Factors of Some Foods

| Food | Sodium (mg) | Potassium (mg) | K-Factor |
|------|-------------|----------------|----------|
| Corn (one 4" cob) | 2 | 196 | 98.00 |
| Cornflakes (1 oz) | 351 | 26 | 0.07 |
| Canned corn (1 oz) | 251 | 166 | 0.70 |
| Chicken (½ breast) | 63 | 220 | 3.50 |
| Fried chicken | 1,220 | 220 | 0.18 |
| Beef (ground sirloin) | 60 | 370 | 6.20 |

| Food | Sodium (mg) | Potassium (mg) | K-Factor |
|---|---|---|---|
| All-beef frank or sausage | 461 | 71 | 0.15 |
| Beans (⅔ cup) | 3 | 340 | 113.00 |
| Canned beans (⅔ cup) | 300 | 264 | 0.90 |
| Tuna (3.5 oz) | 40 | 263 | 6.60 |
| Canned tuna | 409 | 263 | 0.60 |
| Nabisco Shredded Wheat | 30 | 102 | 3.40 |
| Apple (1 medium) | 1 | 159 | 159.00 |
| Apple pie | 282 | 49 | 0.17 |

## Manage Your K-Factor

The K-factor analysis trumpets a message loud and clear: natural food is good news; processed food is usually bad news, unless the processor is interested in maintaining natural standards, as in the case with Shredded Wheat in Table 23.1. It is simple: eat natural foods, don't use salt in recipes, and the K-factor will take care of itself. That's what makes dietary control of high blood pressure so easy. It's healthier and costs less, so why not?

## Plants Are Different

Since plants don't have the same fluid balance and nerve system as animals, sodium is not as important. Table 23.1 shows that plants usually have K-factors of 100 or more. For example, the K-factor of an apple is 159! So, it's not surprising that anthropologists estimate that thousands of years ago when we were largely vegetarian, our dietary K-factor was over 10 and about 16!

## Our "Sea of Salt"

Salary, the word that describes our income, is derived from two words: "salt and ration." Salt (sodium chloride) was once so scarce it was a medium of exchange, like gold dust in 1849 in California, or like money today. Sodium (from salt) was scarce in the human diet and potassium was so abundant that human kidneys focused on conserving sodium and chloride (the two elements of table salt) and were passive to potassium because it was so plentiful. Now salt is so plentiful that we use it to melt ice on sidewalks, and we use too much of it in preparing food. However, kidneys haven't changed.

Table salt is sodium chloride; the same stuff your kidneys work so hard to excrete. Most Americans get from 7 to 10 grams of it daily. That's from 3 to 5 grams of sodium! It doesn't sound like much, but we need a minimum of only 200 milligrams of sodium daily, and the government says a safe and effective range is 1,100 to 3,000 milligrams or 1 to 3 grams. Since salt, sodium chloride, is just under 40 percent sodium, 7 to 10 grams of salt is an enormous amount of sodium compared with the requirement. This excess simply obliterates the K-factor of 3 and reduces it to less than 1!

Table 23.1 shows you why table salt is not the only culprit. Most processed food is excessive in sodium. Compare, for example, the K-factor ratios of beef to hot dogs, or corn to canned corn and cornflakes, and you'll agree that we live in a "sea of salt."

## Are Potassium Supplements Effective?

Some people read about the K-factor and figure out that they could restore potassium-sodium balance by taking potassium supplements. It won't work! The kidneys must still eliminate the excess sodium chloride, and in many people that causes high blood pressure.

Potassium supplements can also cause serious intestinal problems, so people with IBD would create even more problems for themselves. Potassium supplements are prescribed when people are on diuretic medication or have low levels of potassium, but they're not effective to simply restore balance to a poor diet.

The only solution to inadequate potassium is correct food selection. Table 23.2 shows you that natural foods are fine and gives some examples of foods that are extra rich in potassium. These foods conveniently provide a natural potassium boost. Use your food diary to make sure these foods are okay for you.

## Table 23.2

**Convenient Natural Foods Rich in Potassium\* (per serving)**

| Food | Potassium | K-Factor |
|------|-----------|----------|
| Avocado | 1,097 | 52 |
| Bamboo shoots | 640 | 128 |
| Broad beans | 456 | 57 |
| Kidney beans | 713 | 178 |
| Lima beans | 955 | 238 |
| Peas | 644 | 72 |
| Potato | 608 | 87 |
| Squash | 445 | 445 |
| Apricot | 313 | 313 |
| Banana | 451 | 451 |
| Dried lychee | 1,110 | 370 |
| Orange | 250 | 250 |
| Papaya | 780 | 98 |
| Raisins | 751 | 63 |

\*All natural foods have a good K-factor, the potassium:sodium ratio. The foods listed here are especially good for potassium. They can be used as "natural" potassium supplements.

## The Dangers of Diarrhea

People with bowel disorders should strive to maintain a K-factor greater than 6. Getting at least 3,000 milligrams of potassium daily is essential, because diarrhea robs the body of potassium and makes the loss worse by causing dehydration. When you get diarrhea, or have watery stools, two things happen: First, you lose water continuously (although you can make it up by simply drinking more). Second, you continuously lose potassium (you can only make up that loss by eating correctly).

## Dehydration and Electrolyte Imbalance: "Be on Your Guard"

Dehydration and electrolyte imbalance first show up as a lack of energy and fatigue. If they get worse, dizzy spells, fainting spells, and disorientation result. For most people it never goes beyond the statements "I feel so tired. I can't get moving," or "I've had this headache and I feel so tired." In my correspondence with people who have IBD, I noticed that many talk about being "tired" or "lacking energy." While there are many reasons for these feelings, one of them needn't be poor electrolyte balance and chronic borderline dehydration.

If you experience bouts of diarrhea, you've got to be on your guard. Table 23.2 lists foods that are especially rich in potassium. The banana, if fully ripe, is a favorite that can be tolerated by many people with bowel disorders (see Chapter Two). Eat plenty of them. Be sure to always drink water.

## High Blood Pressure: Long-term Potassium-Sodium Imbalance

High blood pressure is called the silent killer because it develops so slowly that most people don't know they've got it until the doctor tells them. No one dies of high blood pressure, but people die of its complications, such as stroke, heart attack, and kidney failure. High blood pressure causes failing eyesight that can lead to blindness, and even a red bulbous nose and flushed face that can ruin good looks. Medications used to control high blood pressure have many unwanted side effects, and they're complicated even more by medications used for IBD or any other inflammatory disease.

And yet dietary control of high blood pressure is very effective. Almost 90 percent of people with high blood pressure can reverse it and maintain control with diet alone.

## Measuring Blood Pressure

Blood pressure is measured with two numbers: *diastolic*, the pressure that remains between heart beats, and *systolic*, the pressure when the heart contracts and pushes the blood into the arteries. Systolic is normally about 40 millimeters (35 to 45 on average) higher than diastolic, so blood pressure is conveniently expressed as systolic over diastolic. For example, normal blood pressure is 120 systolic and 80 diastolic millimeters of mercury. It is conveniently expressed simply as systolic over diastolic, or 120 over 80.

Blood pressure is expressed as millimeters of mercury because it was originally measured by how high it raised a column of mercury. The instrument used to measure blood pressure is called a sphygmomanometer. Your doctor's sphygmomanometer might use a mercury-filled column, but more modern instruments measure with an electronic, battery-operated sphygmomanometer.

## When Is Blood Pressure Too High?

When diastolic exceeds 84, you should be concerned. When it's regularly about 130 over 85, you'd better make serious dietary changes. Even though that level is at the high end of normal and hasn't quite crossed over into the danger zone, it's so close that you'd better take it seriously. At 140 over 90, the doctor will usually take special notice and give advice like "lose weight" and "stop using salt." He or she might even prescribe a diuretic to help lower it by eliminating sodium. At 130 over 85, your life will be about 10 percent shorter, on average, than that of someone whose blood pressure is 110 over 70. At 140 over 100 your probability of an early death is twice that of someone with normal blood pressure. Even at 130 over 85, it makes most other health problems worse.

## Heredity

Heredity has an influence in cases of high blood pressure, but it isn't the same as getting blue eyes from your mother or a hooked nose from your father. You inherit the tendency, but dietary and lifestyle factors you control (or more probably don't control) *cause* high blood pressure. Let me take you through the essential causes.

## The Causes of High Blood Pressure

*Medication* can cause high blood pressure. Drugs used to control inflammation stop the "bad" prostaglandin production to suppress inflammation. Unfortunately, this prostaglandin, in small quantities, helps modulate blood pressure. The plan to control an angry gut will reduce your need for medication, so you can probably avoid this effect.

*Salt* can cause high blood pressure. The sodium in excessive salt use upsets a natural balance between sodium and potassium. The other half of salt, chloride, also has a bad effect on blood pressure, especially in people of African origin, because their kidneys are also more sensitive to chloride. That's why reducing high blood pressure by diet or medication always involves controlling salt.

*Excess weight* causes high blood pressure in two ways. First, each pound of fat needs about 5 miles of capillaries (small vessels through which the heart must pump blood) and it follows that the heart must use more pressure to push all that blood through those capillaries. Worse yet, the extra flab means more insulin is needed to cope with blood sugar. Excess insulin forces the kidneys to elevate the blood pressure. Both reasons lead to one simple dictum: Get your weight down!

## Read Ingredients Lists

Controlling blood pressure means you must rule out any processed food with salt on the ingredients list. Follow that rule even if the processor makes it sound okay by calling it low or moderate sodium. If salt appears on the ingredients list, don't use the product!

The odds that you can control your blood pressure by diet alone are 90 percent. If your investment odds were that good, you'd be rich beyond your wildest dreams.

# CHAPTER 24

# *Fitness*

## As the Twig Is Bent, So Grows the Tree

While exercise reduces the risk of cancer and heart disease and promotes general good health at all ages, the benefits show up mostly after middle age. For both sexes, exercise reduces most cancer and heart disease risk and is especially important in sex-related cancers. In men, prostate cancer risk reduction is related to the effect of exercise on testosterone levels. In women, it affects estrogen in a similar way to reduce breast and ovarian cancer. The more body fat you have the less efficient your body is at handling these hormones, and exercise is the best way to increase lean body mass (muscle) and reduce body fat. Regular exercise is the simplest activity anyone can follow to prevent disease and improve longevity.

## What Kind of Exercise and Why

When you exercise vigorously, do you feel hot? Do you sweat? (I forgot, women perspire and only men sweat.) Notice how your heart beats faster? Ever wonder why?

The answers to these questions are simple. During exercise, your body core temperature increases by a couple of degrees. If I could stick a thermometer inside your muscle—ouch—you would notice a rise of about 2 degrees. That might not seem like much, but it translates to a metabolic rate increase of about 35 percent! That's a lot! Perspiring is your body's attempt to cool itself down, since evaporating sweat takes away heat. An increased pulse rate means your heart is pumping faster to get blood (oxygen) to the muscles.

Notice I said vigorous exercise during which you perspire—that is another way of saying aerobic exercise. Aerobic means with air; anaerobic means without air. You still breathe during anaerobic exercise such as weight lifting, but unless you pump the weights up and down rapidly for a long time, you don't raise your pulse rate enough to elevate your metabolism and cause hard breathing.

Aerobic exercise works the large muscle groups, such as the arms and legs, and also involves other muscle groups in the abdomen and back. This challenges your cardiovascular system to supply sufficient oxygen (aerobic) to make energy for your muscles. Your heart rises to the occasion by increasing its rate—you then breathe more rapidly and deeply to get the necessary oxygen to your muscles.

Aerobic exercise is steady exercise for a long duration, while anaerobic exercise is for a short duration. A comparison helps you see the difference quickly.

Aerobic exercise, such as running, brisk walking, and cycling, will elevate metabolism for a sustained period, say twenty to sixty minutes. This is called a "training effect," because it is training your cardiovascular system to meet the demands and build its muscles. Jogging requires a minimum of fifteen minutes, while a brisk walk should be done for at least twenty-five minutes. These times are determined by how long it takes your heart to reach and maintain a training rate.

A good contrast to a twenty- or thirty-minute jog is to run a 100-yard (or meter) dash. You finish in less than twenty to thirty seconds but find yourself gasping for air for about three minutes at the finish line. The reason you gasp is that your muscles produced the energy for the dash by using energy reserves that don't require air. This creates an energy debt that must be repaid, and it calls for oxygen to regenerate the high energy reserves—this leaves you gasping.

An analogy in everyday life would be running to catch a bus, or quickly running up stairs. The gasping for breath afterward is simply your body demanding repayment of the oxygen debt you created. Your body can handle these anaerobic oxygen-debt incidents better if you exercise anaerobically on a regular basis. The aerobic exercise builds better all-around capacity, even for anaerobic exercise.

## What's Best for You?

Aerobic exercise brings to mind the saying: "Different strokes for different folks." The best exercises for you are the ones you will do regularly. Notice I used the plural. This is because you should vary your regular exercise and work different muscle groups. For example, jog and cycle when the weather is nice and use an indoor rowing machine when it is inclement. Table 24.1 lists some aerobic exercises with the times required to get a good effect.

### Table 24.1

### Aerobic Exercise Programs

| 30 Minutes | 50 Minutes |
| --- | --- |
| Jogging, road or machine | Brisk walk |
| Cross-country skiing, snow or machine | Sensible bicycling or |
| Rowing, on water or machine | stationary cycling |
| Aerobic stepping or dancing | In-line skating |
| Mini-trampoline | Swimming |
| Stair stepping | |

Obviously there are many other devices and methods, so there is something for everyone—no excuses. Don't use motorized devices, with the exception of jogging machines; they don't have the same training effect because your energy output is reduced by the motor. The jogging machine works because it's just the road that's moving and you're keeping up.

## Sports Count

A good active sport also helps to keep you fit. You simply need to use some common sense. Brisk sets of tennis with active opponents are good exercise. In contrast, golf is one way to ruin a good walk; and if you're serious about winning, it increases frustration. Think of racquetball, volleyball, downhill skiing, soccer, basketball, and other sports that increase your pulse for more than thirty minutes and have you perspiring. They count.

## Weight Workouts

Working with weights has a very important place in total body fitness. Sensible weight workouts convert body fat to body muscle. Muscle has a higher metabolic rate and contributes to body fitness. The best way to pursue a weight program is at a fitness center, with a knowledgeable trainer, who can monitor a clear objective of toning muscles, or "bulking up," if that's your objective.

## Overweight or Overfat

Two of the most frustrating things people can do is to look to fashion models (male or female) for a self-image and look up their weight on a height and weight chart. Neither one presents a practical goal. During this century, fashion models have become taller and thinner. Since photographs tend to make us look heavier than we are, designers use tall, skinny models to show their clothes. So, the image we're presented with is moving further and further from reality because our average weight keeps creeping up.

Weight and height charts compiled from life insurance

statistics are in concert with the fashion image. They express an "ideal" weight as a function of height and are based on statistics of who lives longest. They impart the message that being overweight isn't good. Charts that show average weight and height are somewhat more reasonable and impart a more realistic image. Other charts require you to decide whether you have a small, medium, or large frame and go from there. That works a little better, but too often you may have combination frames—broad hips and narrow shoulders, and so on. No person is simply one single type, not even models. That's why the tests that follow are important.

## Body-fat Test

Body-fat composition is the only truly precise index of overweight. Most experts agree that our body-fat content becomes a sort of "set point" that we subconsciously strive to maintain. We have to work hard to lower this set point and then keep it down. The upper level of body fat is 22 percent for women and 15 percent for men. You are better off if your body fat is about 13 percent for men and 20 percent for women. Top athletes usually have much lower levels—down to less than 10 percent—but that's too low for average people.

Determining body fat is routine nowadays. It is done by being weighed underwater and out of water. Because fat floats, it is easy to determine your body fat by subtracting water weight from dry weight. Then divide your fat weight by your dry weight and multiply the decimal by 100 to get your percentage of body fat. You can do it yourself but you will need waterproof scales. Just wear the same bathing suit in and out of the water. If the pool is not deep, simply ball up or squat down on the scale.

## The Float Test

As an alternative to the underwater test, you can estimate your body fat by testing how well you float in a pool. Float on your back and blow all the air out of your lungs, then note what happens.

25 percent fat: You will float.

22 percent fat: You can just stay afloat with shallow breathing.

20 percent fat: You cannot stay afloat without moving your hands or feet.

15 percent fat: You will sink slowly, even with lungs filled with air.

13 percent fat: You will sink readily, even if your lungs are filled with air.

Men should strive for a body composition that sinks readily. Women should strive for a body composition that sinks slowly when they exhale.

Body fat can also be determined with body calipers, used to pinch you in various places, and a weight-height table that gives a value for body fat. You can do this "pinch test" yourself using the directions supplied when you purchase the calipers; they're a good investment.

If you are overfat but not overweight, you know that all you have to do is convert some fat to muscle by exercising regularly. However, if you're both overfat and overweight, you'll need to lose the extra pounds and exercise to build more muscle and bones.

As I explained, if you are overweight, it's because your body is overfat. Or conversely, your lean body mass is too low for your weight. Lean body mass (LBM) is your muscles, bones, and other tissues that have no fat. So when you are overfat, you have to increase muscle size or lose some fat or do both.

If your body composition is right, your weight will be correct for your height and build. For average people who work and maintain a good level of fitness, 15 percent fat is about right for men and 22 percent fat is the upper limit for women. Your LBM should be 85 percent of body weight for men and 78 percent for women. Let's take a 5-foot-6-inch woman at various times in her life, and assume she keeps her weight at 130 pounds.

## Table 24.2

### Weight Distribution

| Age | Total Weight | % Fat | % LBM | Ideal Weight |
|-----|--------------|-------|-------|--------------|
| 20  | 130 lb       | 22    | 78    | 130 lb       |
| 35  | 130 lb       | 26    | 74    | 123 lb       |
| 45  | 130 lb       | 28    | 72    | 120 lb       |

At age 20, this woman was in college, "on the go," active in sports and always busy. At 35, she had become a housewife with two children. While her weight was fine at age 20, according to the charts she was overweight at age 35 and more overweight at age 45 when the children were grown up and she had more time to relax. Even though she has been conscientious and gained no weight, she has noticed an increase in her hips, buttocks, thighs, and under her arms. She feels fat, even though the scale says she is the same weight.

This woman faces a dilemma. She has been very careful not to gain weight, and yet we are saying she is overfat. What can she do?

She can either lose fat or increase muscle mass. Her best course is to do both. The healthy way is for her to drop a little fat and increase muscle mass. Losing fat will increase her life expectancy by reducing her risk of cancer and heart disease. Gaining muscle mass will prevent brittle bones as she gets older. More important, more LBM will increase her basal metabolism.

Fat tissue doesn't require energy; it is stored energy. Thus the BMR of fat is very low. Let's look at the BMR of a woman at three different ages—20, 35, and 45—who doesn't watch her weight and body-fat composition.

## Table 24.3

### Results of Losing LBM

| Age | Total Weight | LBM (lb) | Fat (lb) | % Fat | BMR (calories) |
|-----|-------------|----------|----------|-------|----------------|
| 20 | 130 lb | 101 | 29 | 22 | 1,339 |
| 35 | 135 lb | 96 | 39 | 28 | 1,331 |
| 45 | 140 lb | 94 | 46 | 33 | 1,294 |

You will notice that her total BMR declines in proportion to her lean body mass; as she loses LBM, she also reduces the calories she needs to stay alive.

Muscle is active tissue; it's always burning calories. Fat is inactive; it doesn't require calories and it reduces BMR calories. Excess fat is added under the skin first, where it insulates and retains heat and therefore reduces the BMR needed to keep us warm. Consequently, BMR declines even more than in the above example.

Your lean body mass is like the engine in your car. The gas you burn depends mostly on the size of the engine, not the size of your car. Gas mileage for a loaded car is about the same as for an empty car until you load it up to the point where you have the engine running at full speed just to make it go. Heavy people spend even less energy exercising than you would expect from the extra weight they carry. It is because their lean body mass, like the car engine, is smaller and well insulated to save heat. So they get by with even less energy than a person with the same LBM, but without the fat. Research has shown that overweight people learn to get through life with less energy. They learn to move more slowly—find the least energetic route by taking the bus—and when they participate in sports, they learn to use less motion than lean people. It's called adaptation!

## Everyone Can Exercise

I have worked with many people in my career, and without exception, I have learned that everyone can exercise. If you've got a chronic illness like IBD, you will have to search for an exercise that works for you, but a little searching and asking an expert will put you on the road to fitness.

Most people avoid exercise by not finding time. Again, I have never met a single person who couldn't find the time. I personally found that the only way I could find time to exercise regularly was to get up an hour earlier every day. It worked, and I never missed a session unless I decided to take the day off—it was my decision.

Statistics prove that people who decide to exercise after work are more likely to quit than people who exercise before work. It simply confirms that life is complex and time is at a premium. You should put the highest premium on your health, so exercise to achieve fitness.

# CHAPTER 25

# *Outlook*

Why is it that when I interview people with IBD, I meet some who are incredibly successful? They have enviable incomes, beautiful families, and are the general picture of success. I notice that these people have varying degrees of IBD—with some it is terrible and with others it is mild—which is no different from all the others I meet with the disease. However, one characteristic is quite different: their outlooks. They hardly talk about their illnesses, and if I didn't ask questions, I wouldn't know anything about their problems.

In contrast, those who wax long and often about the difficulties of life with IBD generally are not nearly as successful. It is quite possible that the stressful nature of the disease is something some people have difficulty dealing with; consequently, they become somewhat focused on the disease rather than other aspects of their lives. This difference in attitudes reminds me of a sociological study conducted on twin brothers. One story stood out.

Identical twin boys were born to a couple who, experts agreed, should never have lived together, let alone had children. The boys' father, an unskilled worker with no obvious ambition, never held a steady job. He drank heavily, lived from day to day, and had no goals. The mother did menial tasks intermittently, when she could get work. Both parents drank excessively and often lived on welfare. Both boys were raised as much by neighbors and each other as by their parents. By the age of 10, they were left almost to raise themselves.

Survival was the word that described their home life. Their parents fought so violently at times that police were called to stop the arguments; sometimes they had to sleep off their alcoholic condition at the police station. Both parents regularly beat the children and used words like "damn kids" or "no-good kids." The boys' home life wasn't the foundation of a good outlook.

By age 35, the twin boys were a contrast in success. Tom was an unskilled worker and drank heavily, not unlike his parents. He didn't hold jobs very long, fought with his wife, and the local police knew him quite well. Tom and his wife lived in the same squalid environment where they had grown up. They were well known to the welfare authorities and learned to take advantage of everything the government would provide.

Jim was the complete opposite. He had worked hard at menial part-time jobs while going to school at night and on weekends. He saved what little money he could and, when he finished school, started a small business. At age 35, his small company was growing, and he was becoming a wealthy man. His family life was also rewarding. He and his lovely wife worked together to raise their two small children in a harmonious atmosphere. Their modest home was neat, clean, and expressed pride of ownership. They were a close, happy family, enjoyed life, and were serious about their future.

As part of the study, a social worker interviewed both brothers and asked them exactly the same questions. Curiously, she got exactly the same answer to one pertinent question: "Why did you become what you are today?" The answer was: "What else could I do growing up in that place?"

Each man had exactly the same lack of opportunity, and each one had a vision of himself. Tom saw himself as nothing. Jim saw himself as a person who had no place to go but up. The only difference between the brothers was how they got from where they were to where they visualized themselves. For Tom, it was easy—do nothing. For Jim, it required commitment to an objective. Tom said to himself: "This is what life is like." Jim said to himself: "I can always do better than this."

## The Power of Visualization

A sculptor once explained how she could take a block of stone and make a beautiful statue: "The statue is already there; all I do is chip away the extra stone, then smooth and polish what is left." When pressed a little further, she explained more fully: "Before I visualize the figure in the statue, I get to know the stone. Stone has a complex texture shaped over millions of years by the elements. Once I understand the character of the stone, the figure inside is clear and can be unlocked and live forever in harmony with the elements that created the stone."

We can take a lesson from the sculptor and the twin boys. Forces that we don't control start to shape and build the texture of our character before we are even aware of ourselves. These forces include heredity, home life, the environment in which we grow—everything around us. They form the fabric that will emerge as character.

We constantly call on all this texture to visualize our lives and shape the future. As time passes, more and more of the stone of life is chipped away and parts of each individual statue get finished. So long as we are alive, there is always time to be better and increase the abundance of life. The better we live in harmony with the world around us, the smoother the texture becomes.

Nothing can be accomplished without a vision. Let the vision of your future become your objective, just like Tom and Jim did, but never sell yourself short. Only two factors separate success from failure: vision and perseverance.

Education doesn't create success, nor does physical beauty.

Parents can't make you succeed either. They can all help, but only you can create success. Success means visualizing a general goal and reshaping it as you get closer, until you achieve it.

Ask yourself a simple, but clear question: "What is success for me?" Recognize that the answer will change, probably annually when you are young and even less frequently as you mature. Notice I said "mature," not age. You can be mature at age 20, but not old until 80; or old and mature at age 20. I know people over 90 who still talk about the future. It gets back to success and goals.

## Goal Setting

Goals should be realistic but require that you stretch your capability. They should take into account your resources, but more important, your potential. Focus on the fundamentals:

- *Love:* We need to love and be loved. People who experience a loving relationship live better and longer. One objective should focus on building a lasting relationship based on love and respect. For most people, this is marriage and the family, but it can be—or include—other relationships.
- *Health objectives:* Never compromise on what you can become. Be as healthy as you can be, no matter what your physical qualities.
- *Respect:* Success with people and in commerce usually depends on just one word: respect. It starts with yourself and applies to everyone you meet.
- *Career objectives:* Not money! Career objectives should focus on achievements and should include milestones to measure progress.

Other goals depend on what is important in your life. If you have small children, you should set some goals about helping them achieve their potentials, their attitudes about health, friends, love, respect, and setting the right ideals for a bright future.

## Dare to Take Chances

Everything about life is a series of risks from the instant of conception to the hour of death. Often the only thing that separates success from failure is the willingness to dare. It can be summarized in the following poem:

### *To Dare*

To laugh is to risk appearing the fool.
To weep is to risk appearing sentimental.
To reach for another is to risk involvement.
To expose your ideas, your dreams before a crowd is
　to risk their loss.
To love is to risk not being loved in return.
To live is to risk dying.
To believe is to risk failure.

Risks must be taken, because the greatest hazard in life is to risk nothing. People who don't risk avoid suffering and sorrow, but they cannot learn, feel, change, grow, love, and live. Chained by their attitudes, they are slaves; they have forfeited freedom. Only a person who risks is free.

## Basic Good Habits

Bad habits bring instant rewards; good habits take a long time for their payout. A smoker is instantly gratified with a mild "high," but a nonsmoker might never know that his health is superior. However, sooner or later, the good habits of a clean lifestyle do pay rewards.

Basic good habits are simple:

- Diet
- Lifestyle

- Integrity
- Loving yourself and others
- Respecting yourself and others
- Caring relationships

## Strive

If you don't use it, you lose it. This summarizes everything about life from your mental capacity to your athletic ability.

Success is what you do when no one is looking. Sound strange? It isn't. Successful people work hard when they are alone and no one is looking. It is why the concert pianist practices after the concert is over, the writer is up working at 5:00 A.M., or the successful athlete goes alone to a quiet field and hones his or her skill. These people learn to grade themselves. Their teachers and coaches are guides to help them discover the limits of their capabilities, but it is inner drive that makes them work when no one is looking; thus they build the capacity for success.

## So You've Got IBD

Even though you have IBD, let it help you to understand that pain and hardship can be overcome. Let it energize you to be like the athlete or musician who practices alone to improve his or her skills and get better. Use this challenge to set an objective to achieve a level of health that will make you a leader among people with IBD. Commit to good health and your life's goals so you can set an example for others with the disease. Just remember that Dwight D. Eisenhower led the greatest crusade in history and became President of the United States—and he had Crohn's disease!

# References

## Preface

Saibil, Fred. 1997. *Crohn's Disease and Ulcerative Colitis: Everything You Need to Know.* New York: Firefly Books.

Thompson, W. Grant. 1993. *Coping with Colitis and Crohn's Disease.* New York: Plenum Press.

Scala, James. 1998. *The New Arthritis Relief Diet.* New York: Plume.

Janowitz, Henry D. 1989. *Your Gut Feelings.* New York: Oxford University Press.

## Chapter Two: Putting People's Experiences into Food

Reif, S., et al. 1997. Pre-illness Dietary Factors in Inflammatory Bowel Disease. *Gut* 40(6): 754–60.

Candy, S., et al. 1995. The Value of an Elimination Diet in the Management of Patients with Ulcerative Colitis. *South African Medical Journal* 85(11): 1176–9.

Probert, C. S., et al. 1996. Diet of South Asians with Inflammatory Bowel Disease. *Arquivos de Gastroenterologia* 33(3): 132–5.

Zorich, N. L., et al. 1997. A Randomized, Double-blind Study of the Effect of Olestra on Disease Activity in Patients with Quiescent Inflammatory Bowel Disease. Olestra in IBD Study Group. *American Journal of Medicine* 103(5): 389–99.

Afdhal, N. H., et al. 1989. Remission Induction in Refractory Crohn's Disease Using a High Calorie Whole Diet. *Journal of Parenteral and Enteral Nutrition* 13(4): 362–5.

## Chapter Six: Do's, Don'ts, and Cautions of Food Selection

Pennington, Jean A. 1989. *Bowes and Church's Food Values of Portions Commonly Used*, 15th ed. Philadelphia: J. B. Lippincott Co.

## Chapter Eight: Medicinal Foods

O'Sullivan, M. A., and C. A. O'Morain. 1998. Nutritional Therapy in Crohn's Disease. *Inflammatory Bowel Disease* 4(1): 45–53.

Hunter, J. O. 1998. Nutritional Factors in Inflammatory Bowel Disease. *European Journal Gastroenterology and Hepatology* 10(3): 235–7.

O'Morain, C. A. 1987. Nutritional Therapy in Ambulatory Patients. *Digestive Diseases and Sciences* 32(12 Suppl): 95S–99S.

Teahon, K., et al. 1995. Alterations in Nutritional Status and Disease Activity During Treatment of Crohn's Disease with Elemental Diet. *Scandanavian Journal of Gastroenterology* 30(1): 54–60.

## Chapter Nine: People Who Don't Get Inflammatory Diseases

Kromann, N., and A. Green. 1980. Epidemiological Studies in the Upernavik District, Greenland. *Acta Medica Scandanavica* 208: 401–6.

Horrobin, D. F. 1987. Low Prevalence of Coronary Heart Disease, Psoriasis, Asthma, and Rheumatoid Arthritis in Eskimos: Are They Caused by High Dietary Intake of Eicosapentaenoic Acid, a Genetic Variation of Essential Fatty Acid Metabolism, or a Combination of Both? *Medical Hypotheses* 22: 421–8.

Recht, L., et al. 1990. Hand Handicap and Rheumatoid Arthritis in a Fish-eating Society (the Faeroe Islands). *Journal of Internal Medicine* 227: 49–55.

Cathcart, E. S., and W. A. Gonnerman. 1991. Fish Oil Fatty

Acids and Experimental Arthritis. *Rheumatic Diseases Clinics of North America* 17: 235–42.

Spiller, Gene A., and James Scala, eds. 1989. *New Protective Roles for Selected Nutrients*. New York: Alan R. Liss. Omega-3 Fatty Acids: Epidemiological and Clinical Aspects; 5: 229–52.

Buhner, S., et al. 1994. Ileal and Colonic Fatty Acid Profiles in Patients with Active Crohn's Disease. *Gut* 35(10): 1424–28.

Siguel, E. N., and R. H. Lerman. 1996. Prevalence of Essential Fatty Acid Deficiency in Patients with Chronic Gastrointestinal Disorders. *Metabolism* 45(1): 12–23.

Prikazska, M. and R. Simoncic. 1997. Nutrition and Crohn's Disease. *Bratislavske Lekarske Listy* 98(2): 107–10.

Hunter, J. O. 1998. Nutritional Factors in Inflammatory Bowel Disease. *European Journal of Gastroenterology and Hepatology* 10(3): 235–7.

Kuroki, F., et al. 1997. Serum n3 Polyunsaturated Fatty Acids Are Depleted in Crohn's Disease. *Digestive Diseases and Sciences* 42(6): 1137–41.

## Chapter Eleven: Clinical Research Results: Inflammation Can Be Managed

Belluzzi, A., et al. 1994. Effects of New Fish Oil Derivative on Fatty Acid Phospholipid-membrane Pattern in a Group of Crohn's Disease Patients. *Digestive Diseases and Sciences* 39(12): 2589–94.

Lorenz-Meyer, H., et al. 1996. Omega-3 Fatty Acids and Low Carbohydrate Diet for Maintenance of Remission in Crohn's Disease. *Scandanavian Journal of Gastroenterology* 31(8): 778–85.

Shoda, R., et al. 1995. Therapeutic Efficacy of N-3 Polyunsaturated Fatty Acid in Experimental Crohn's Disease. *Journal Gastroenterology* 30 Suppl. 8: 98–101.

Ikehata, A., et al. 1992. Effect of Intravenously Infused Eicosapentaenoic Acid on the Leukotriene Generation in Patients with Active Crohn's Disease. *American Journal of Clinical Nutrition* 56(5): 938–42.

Marotta, F., et al. 1995. Shark Fin Enriched Diet Prevents

Mucosal Lipid Abnormalities in Experimental Acute Colitis. *Digestion* 56(1): 46–51.

Belluzzi, A., et al. 1996. Effect of an Enteric-coated Fish-oil Preparation on Relapses in Crohn's Disease. *New England Journal of Medicine* 334(24): 1557–60.

Buhner, S., et al. 1994. Ileal and Colonic Fatty Acid Profiles in Patients with Active Crohn's Disease. *Gut* 35(10): 1424–28.

Campbell, J. M., et al. 1997. Metabolic Characteristics of Healthy Adult Males as Affected by Ingestion of a Liquid Nutritional Formula Containing Fish Oil, Oligosaccharides, Gum Arabic and Antioxidant Vitamins. *Food and Chemical Toxicology* 35(12): 1165–76.

Vilaseca, J., et al. 1990. Dietary Fish Oil Reduces Progression of Chronic Inflammatory Lesions in a Rat Model of Granulomatous Colitis. *Gut* 31(5): 539–44.

French, M. A., et al. 1997. Polyunsaturated Fat in the Diet May Improve Intestinal Function in Patients with Crohn's Disease. *Biochimica et Biophysica Acta* 1360(3): 262–70.

### Chapter Twenty-two: Calcium: A Case for Strong Bones

Sowers, MF. R., et al. 1998. Prevalence of Renal Stones in a Population-based Study with Dietary Calcium, Oxalate, and Medical Exposures. *American Journal of Epidemiology* 147(10): 914–20.

### Chapter Twenty-four: Fitness

Ballard-Barbash, R., and C. A. Swanson. 1996. Body Weight: Estimation of Risk for Breast and Endometrial Cancers. *American Journal of Clinical Nutrition* (Mar.) 63(3 Suppl.): 437S–441S.

Ursin, G., et al. 1995. Early Adult Body Weight, Body Mass Index, and Premenopausal Bilateral Breast Cancer: Data from a Case-Control Study. *Breast Cancer Research and Treatment* 33(1): 75–82.

Thune, I., et al. 1997. Physical Activity and the Risk of Breast Cancer. *New England Journal of Medicine* (May 1) 336(18): 1269–75.

# Index